YOUR PRIMAL BODY

YOUR PRIMAL BODY

The Paleo Way to Living Lean,
Fit, and Healthy at Any Age

Mikki Reilly, MFS, CSCS

Da Capo
LIFE
LONG

A Member of the Perseus Books Group

Designed by Pauline Brown
Set in 11.5 point Warnock Pro Light by the Perseus Books Group

Cataloging-in-Publication data for this book is
available from the Library of Congress.

First Da Capo Press edition 2013
ISBN: 978-0-7382-1637-9

Published by Da Capo Press
A Member of the Perseus Books Group
www.dacapopress.com

Note: The information in this book is true and complete to the best of our
knowledge. This book is intended only as an informative guide for those wishing
to know more about health issues. In no way is this book intended to replace,
countermand, or conflict with the advice given to you by your own physician.
The ultimate decision concerning care should be made between you and your
doctor. We strongly recommend you follow his or her advice. Information in
this book is general and is offered with no guarantees on the part of the authors
or Da Capo Press. The authors and publisher disclaim all liability in connection
with the use of this book. The names and identifying details of people associated
with events described in this book have been changed. Any similarity to actual
persons is coincidental.

Da Capo Press books are available at special discounts for bulk purchases in the
U.S. by corporations, institutions, and other organizations. For more
information, please contact the Special Markets Department at the
Perseus Books Group, 2300 Chestnut Street, Suite 200, Philadelphia, PA, 19103,
or call (800) 810-4145, ext. 5000, or e-mail special.markets@perseusbooks.com.

10 9 8 7 6 5 4 3 2 1

Contents

Foreword

Mikki Reilly has done something unique with what I and others have been calling the *evolutionary* or Paleo approach to diet and fitness. She, in essence, has written the "user's manual" that takes the theory and applies it practically to exercise and lifestyle—it's the "how-to" for Paleo followers.

She's been able to do this because of her excellent background and professional credentials—she earned the highly esteemed certified strength and conditioning specialist (CSCS) credential from the National Strength and Conditioning Association (NSCA) and the master of fitness sciences (MFS) from the International Sports Sciences Association (ISSA). But even more because she is a fitness trainer who has been in the trenches, so to speak, working with clients daily to see how an evolutionary approach is altering lives. Her clients of all ages got stronger and leaner by changing their diet and performing functional, high-intensity exercise, and in this book you will read their stories. I've long asserted from personal experience that "chronic cardio" was not the way to go, and now we have a blueprint for the kind of exercise that takes the best advantage of our natural gene expression—laid out and made simple for everyday use.

When I first began writing about the Paleo approach back in 1995, few people were interested. But that has changed. Following the diet and lifestyle of our earliest ancestors, who were around for over 2 million years and lived fitter, healthier lives in many ways than we do today, is appealing to more and more people. Mikki has made it all the more accessible to do, and just in time, as now women are showing interest, and she is a unique model for how a woman can embrace the Paleo way. In fact, I might go so far as to call her the "female face of Paleo," inspiring other women, as well as everyone, to adopt a more natural, healthy way of life that puts an end to fads and fashion in fitness.

A simple fact today's scientists have discovered is that we humans evolved as hunter-gathers, moving and eating in specific ways that shaped us genetically and had us survive. Not only survive, but thrive! The latest evidence shows that our ancestors lived out their days relatively disease free and with bodies that equaled those of our modern-day Olympic athletes. *Your Primal Body* shows us how you can do what they did, and combined with our modern environment, thrive even better.

Arthur De Vany, PhD
Author, *The New Evolution Diet: What Our Paleolithic Ancestors Can Teach Us About Weight Loss, Fitness, and Aging*

Introduction

The book you hold in your hands, *Your Primal Body: The Paleo Way to Living Lean, Fit, and Healthy at Any Age,* is a doorway to the total transformation of your body, your health, and your life. It's about fitness, but unlike most fitness books today, this book offers more than directions and a routine for changing your body. It gives you a revolutionary new context for weight loss, pain-free movement, building muscle, heart health, and longevity—all based on scientific information about humans that are 2.6 million years old.

The program you will read about in this book is unique in one main way: It's based on your DNA. Because the human genome has not changed in the last forty thousand years, you want to mimic what the earliest humans did that worked. Their DNA was shaped over 2.6 million years since they came down from the trees to begin a lifestyle of hunting and gathering. The environment they encountered was one that built strong muscles and lean bodies, so they could survive the harsh conditions that prevailed for eons. When you exercise and eat according to the lifestyles of the earliest humans, you gain a host of advantages that were honed over millennia to keep you in top condition.

My plan also includes a fitness program based on doing what your DNA has programmed your body to do. The old model, still used in most gyms and programs today, requires endless hours of cardio, boring low-fat diets, and machine-dependent strength training. The low-fat, aerobic approach has been around for decades, ever since Kenneth Cooper wrote *Aerobics* in the late '60s and Jane Fonda put millions of women on the aerobic dance floor in the '70s. But now, there's a new trend in town. My 5-Step Primal Body Program, the backbone of this book, will turn your world upside down and change forever how you think about fitness. Dr. Cooper; move over; Jane Fonda, move over; and yes, Jillian Michaels, move over, too. The biggest losers are about to become the biggest winners, and working out just got a whole lot more fun.

The 5-Step Primal Body Program shows you how to be congruent with your DNA and gives you a step-by-step program to get you in alignment with the way your genes were designed to be expressed. It is based on my twenty years of experience in the trenches, working daily with individuals whose stories you'll read and pictures you'll see in these pages. My approach is not theoretical, nor is it only what I've done for myself—although in this book I include plenty of scientific theory and tell you how I transformed my own body. What makes my experience valuable is that I have helped hundreds of people see remarkable results when their eating and moving patterns become an expression of their human genome.

Fads come and go, most of them based on information designed to appeal to our vanity. Few coaches you'll run into have as their mission restoring our original, genetically programmed state of health and fitness. This, however, has been my purpose and passion, driving me to become highly credentialed as a college-educated, award-winning fitness trainer with an internationally recognized fitness certification—certified strength and conditioning specialist (CSCS) from the National Strength and Conditioning Association, and the master of fitness sciences from the International Sports Sciences Association (ISSA). In addition, I was awarded the Distinguished Achievement Award from ISSA, which signifies placement in the top 1 percent of certified trainers worldwide.

You are in good hands. I am highly qualified to help you change your body. And so are you, by taking advantage of the physiology you've inherited to maintain superior health and fitness—*Your Primal Body*.

HOW TO USE THIS BOOK

This book is divided into three parts. The first two provide a detailed overview of the program (with lots of practical information); the third part helps you put it all together to develop your own Primal Body plan. Here's an outline of what you will find in this book:

Part 1, "The Primal Body—Our Genetic Inheritance" introduces the background of my unique approach and shows how I apply it to health and weight loss. In Chapter 1, you'll read the science behind why our human ancestors had the body of Olympic athletes and learn about their diet and movement patterns. I'll answer all of your questions and challenges about this approach. In Chapter 2, I show how mimicking our ancestors' diet and movement patterns can turn your body into a highly efficient fat-burning machine for the most effective method of fat loss. In Chapter 3, I dispel the notion that aging must be equated with disease and show how the Primal Body Program supports you to become a healthy, active centenarian. I explore how exercise effects gene expression, extending life span beyond what is considered the normal range in our modern society.

Part 2, "The 5-Step Primal Body Program," outlines in five chapters what you must do to get on the evolutionary fitness wagon and ride. Each step includes inspiring, first-person stories of people I worked with who transformed their body by changing over to a Primal lifestyle, and shows you how you can, too. Here's a brief summary of each step:

In "Step One—Eat the Anti-Inflammation Primal Diet," you learn what inflammation is and how this condition becomes chronic due to modern, high-carb diets. Guidelines are given for the kinds of foods that provide a healthy balance of good fats and low-glycemic carbs, aimed at greater weight loss, but also pain-free movement.

In "Step Two—Supplement with the Super Six," I explain why our human ancestors didn't take supplements, but we must. I introduce the "Super Six," my list of supplements to ensure you match the nutrient density our ancestors got from their diet. Each supplement is described in detail for its benefits, and recommended dosages are given.

In "Step Three—Restore Your Muscles to Pain-Free Movement," I show how you can increase mobility and flexibility through the Self-Myofascial Release (SMR) technique. I give instructions based on the seven Primal movements and describe twelve positions for SMR, with model photos included. The result is your body is now ready for strength training and high-intensity interval training, the core of the Primal exercise program.

In "Step Four—Build Muscle with Primal Movement," you learn how to build muscle and burn fat through functional training, rather than by more traditional techniques that require isolating muscles on machines. Functional training, emphasizing movements that are found in daily activities, mimics how our ancestors moved to stay muscular and lean naturally, congruent with their genetic blueprint. I show you how to do this with fourteen illustrated functional training movements.

In "Step Five—Kick Up Your Metabolism to Burn Fat Faster," I explain the surprising news that traditional cardio/aerobic exercise can actually make you fat, while a Primal form of exercise, high-intensity interval training, is more effective for weight loss and all-around conditioning. In this step, I also present clear instructions on safe, effective use of kettlebells (the cannonball-shaped weight with the handle) to crank up your metabolism and firm up your body.

Part 3, "Putting It All Together," brings all the information and techniques described in the 5-Step Primal Body Program together to answer the question "So what do I do now?" In Chapter 9, I provide practical advice about how to start planning and cooking simple meals of mostly protein, fat, and nonstarchy vegetables, with plenty of recipes to get you started. In Chapter 10, I help you design an exercise program, tailor-made to your specific fitness level and immediate goals, using functional strength-training and metabolic activities. In Chapter 11, I show you how to measure your results to maintain lifelong success on the Primal Body Program. I also provide resources for acquiring Primal cooking aids (see page 197), as well as a recommended reading list and bibliography of books on the Primal theory and lifestyle (see page 205).

Your Primal Body is a book and program to mark the beginning of transforming your fitness and health. If you have been following a program that has not produced the results you've wanted, or if you are new to fitness and have never trained or eaten healthily before, the Primal Body Program will get you going in the right direction—the same direction your human genome has been going in over the past few million years.

This is your opportunity to use that evolution to your advantage. Stop struggling to carve out the body you want by going against your genetic blueprint, and join a revolution that takes you home to your original body.

I wish you the best in your adventure to discover *Your Primal Body*.

PART I

The Primal Body:
Our Genetic Inheritance

Chapter 1

Why Our Ancestors Were Right

Jog to burn fat—the longer the better.

Avoid saturated fats to stay healthy.

Eat six meals a day.

Always stretch before training.

Do cardio after weight training.

The list goes on of the conventional wisdom that we've all been led to believe about fitness and weight loss. For the past four decades, since the aerobic exercise revolution got under way, these sacred tenets have kept people doing hours of cardio exercise on a treadmill or bike, sweating the pounds away while sticking to a low-fat diet in an effort to become healthy and fit.

But all of that is changing, and while what's taking its place is very new, it's also very old.

You are about to discover that the way to getting a fit, lean, and healthy body—one that moves powerfully and gracefully at any age—has nothing to do with hours of "chronic cardio," low-fat diets, or using machines to work out in the gym. This is because becoming slim, muscular, and healthy is how you return—in both diet and exercise—to the way that your body was intended to function originally, based on millions of years of evolution and as proven by modern science.

As a personal fitness trainer, working with a wide range of clients—including overweight, middle-aged men and women as well as top-tier athletes—I am bringing a new paradigm of fitness to people that is natural, effective, and fun. My Primal Body Program turns the old, more conventional wisdom on its ear, because it is based on the premise that your body is genetically designed for health and fitness on a scale far superior to what you experience today—even if you consider yourself in good condition. Your body already *is* the Primal Body I am talking about. What you'll find here is a program designed for you to train and eat in ways that are congruent with the body you already have, which has been shaped by the events of 2.6 million years and unchanged over the past forty thousand years.

The Primal Body Program is a path consisting of five steps to realign your lifestyle to fulfill that original genetic design of your body for increased health and longevity. When you embrace the Primal Body Program, you no longer go against your genetic inheritance. You can lose those extra pounds, whether 10 or 100, bring a cut and youthful appearance to your muscles and overall posture, and enjoy sexual vitality throughout your life (and move pain free to maintain a muscular and functioning body in every aspect of your daily life).

Sound like a dream come true? It is, and the surprising news is: *All this is your birthright!* When you express your genes in the way they evolved to be expressed, then all the weight loss, toned muscles, and pain-free ease of movement you've ever wanted is yours—permanently. This is not a miracle but a natural physical state, available to any human being at any age or any level of fitness.

HOW I DISCOVERED MY INNER (AND OUTER) CAVEWOMAN

I've been a personal trainer for twenty years, but in 2002 I went back to school to finish my degree in exercise and health science and communication. It was there that I discovered the research behind what has become known as the Primal theory of fitness, an approach based on how our Paleolithic ancestors moved and ate. I was surprised and then intrigued to learn that this approach closely paralleled what I was already doing to get results for myself and clients.

Over the years, I had tried all kinds of diets in my personal exploration of health and fitness, immersing myself thoroughly in whatever the current approach was. I followed a macrobiotic diet for some time, and then I became a vegetarian for seven years. From there, I went low-fat. I followed the Zone diet made popular by Barry Sears, until I discovered the low-carb Atkins diet.

Dr. Atkins was a low-carb guru in the 1970s who advocated a strict regimen of 20 grams of carbohydrate a day for the first fourteen days of his program. This was designed to put the body into a state of ketosis, in which the body burns ketones as an alternate fuel to glucose (you'll find more info on ketosis on pages 24–25). I had great success with a number of my clients who used this method to lose 30 to 40 pounds.

While working on my degree at the University of California at Santa Barbara, I discovered the Paleo diet, a newer low-carb approach with an emphasis on daily protein and healthy omega-3–rich fats. I began following the work of Dr. Loren Cordain, one of the world's leading experts on the diet of our Stone Age ancestors.

I read everything I could of Dr. Cordain's research (he's written over one hundred peer-reviewed scientific articles on the health benefits of the Stone Age diet for contemporary people), learning of the recent discoveries of paleo-anthropologists that revealed our early human ancestors' lifestyles. It was an eye-opening adventure!

Cordain delved into what archaeologists and paleo-anthropologists were finding about the diet and movement patterns of early humans from their appearance some 2.6 million years ago. From remains that have been found, it is clear that early hunter-gatherers suffered from none of the diseases of modern man, such as heart disease, cancer, diabetes, or obesity; rather, they lived a relatively disease-free life. Whatever our cave-ancestors were doing kept them in an optimal state of fitness and health.

Most important for me was what I had known all along, that a low-carb, high-protein diet with healthy fats was the best way to eat for health and permanent weight loss. Now I had both a context and confirmation for why: It is the ancestral diet we evolved on and therefore is perfectly congruent with our human genome.

ANCIENT GENES AND MODERN HUMANS

The human genome is the set of chromosomes you and I have in every cell of our body—our DNA—giving expression to who we are and how we function. Geneticists have recently mapped the complete human genome, a stunning achievement that is altering what we know about our history as a species. It's been documented that the human genome evolved over a period of 2.6 million years but remained the same since the last forty thousand years—the time period when early humans started to hunt animals and gather vegetables and fruits as a way of life.

In other words, you and I have the same DNA as those Stone Age hunter-gatherers, and we carry in our cells a genetic blueprint that was shaped in an environment very different from the one we experience today. What does this mean for our health and fitness in modern times? Dr. Cordain refers to a rule most biologists agree applies, when he states, "Biological organisms are healthiest when their life circumstances most closely approximate the conditions for which their genes were selected."

The lack of close approximation between modern and ancient has led to a question he and other theorists have started to ask, "Are we modern humans living in a way that is out of step with our inherited genetic design?" They go even further to ask, "Could our genetic 'incongruence' be the reason for the many diseases that plague modern humans, diseases that weren't around back in our ancestors' times?"

Biologists tell us that when early humans radically changed their diet and activity patterns by becoming agriculturists ten thousand years ago, the so-called diseases of civilization—atherosclerosis, cancer, diabetes, arthritis, and others—began to appear. While there is a lively debate afoot in the scientific community about the evidence for this, as reported recently in the *New York Times*,[1] there are no clear signs that these diseases were anywhere near as prominent in Paleolithic times as they have been in more recent evolution, especially since the agricultural revolution.

These questions and the answers I was discovering made sense to me from my own experience. Having eaten a low-carb, high-protein diet for years, I found myself to be in the best physical condition of my life. My weight was easy to maintain and I had plenty of energy to train, both in strength building and in my most recent interest, high-intensity interval exercises. I was definitely doing something right!

I began to be interested in what life was like for our early hunter-gatherer ancestors, and in my research found some fascinating information about how they lived.

STONE AGE LIFESTYLES

Let's take a closer look at the lifestyles of the earliest humans to learn more about how they functioned—in particular, their diet and movement patterns.

By about twelve thousand years ago, hunter-gatherers had moved into most of the habitable regions of the earth. In small, mobile bands, our ancestors adapted to almost all climates and environments, from the Arctic to the tropics, by exploiting whatever resources they found available.

These bands, often comprised of twenty-five to fifty people, moved seasonally to take advantage of different sources of food as they became available. Within the group, women did most of the gathering and men did the hunting, although this gender distinction was not universal. To survive, everyone learned about the geographic area, the food sources, and the dangers, and this knowledge was shared communally. Everyone had to be prepared to act in ways that fended off danger, whether from natural disasters or attacks by predators. Conditions were harsh, but in spite of this, our Stone Age ancestors had a great deal of leisure, enjoying recreational activities, such as singing, dancing, playing instruments, and story-telling around the open fire.

What did the early hunter-gatherer tribes eat? Studies show their diet consisted mainly of animal protein, fats, and limited carbohydrates, such as roots and vegetables pulled from the ground, and fruits plucked from bushes and trees. They ate a variety of plant foods that provided an abundance of vitamins, minerals, antioxidants, and other phytonutrients.

Although there may be some resemblance between the foods they ate and our modern versions of the same foods, most of their foods were very different. Not only is nutrient density greatly diminished in modern food, but the actual chemistry of the food, after centuries of hybrid growing, has been altered almost beyond recognition. For example, the wild game they feasted on was grass-fed, as animals grazed freely before domestication, and it was loaded with the essential fatty acid omega-3, an anti-inflammatory form of fat. This is completely unlike modern cattle, which are grain-fed and therefore produce meat high in the fatty acid omega-6, a pro-inflammatory form of fat. An apple a million years ago had much less sugar in it than the fruit of today and would probably not be appealing to our modern taste for sweetness in fruits.

As I have said, modern humans have the same DNA as early hunter-gatherers did. This is important in light of their lifestyles as compared to ours, because our genes determine our nutritional and physical activity needs. Our modern body is "expecting" to meet with the same foods and activity patterns it had grown accustomed to over the past forty thousand years, a period in which nothing in our human genome changed. The problem is that our diet has changed, especially as we began to grow our food and domesticate animals ten thousand years ago, when grain-based agriculture became a way of life. Archaeologists uncovering remains of early humans tell us that starting around that time, there was a characteristic reduction in body stature, an increase in bone mineral disorders, an increase in the number of dental cavities, and a decrease in the average life span.

Another fact brought to light by recent science is that before the advent of agriculture, humans led much more active lives. Archaeological evidence shows hunter-gatherers to be lean, fit—much like a modern-day athlete—and free from chronic diseases. Exercise was not done during leisure time, as it is today; rather, it was a part of everyday life. Hunting, foraging, escape from predators, water transport, and all of the movements needed to survive in the Paleolithic environment shaped a genetic pattern that survives today.

A further study by Cordain showed that one thing is clear from our understanding of early human ancestors: The genetic model for human physical activity was not developed in the gymnasium or in the sports arena. It was established through adaptive pressures inherent in the environment over millions of years of evolution. When the human body is viewed through this lens, it becomes clear that the conventional thinking about diet and exercise is deeply flawed.

THE COST OF ADAPTATION

Given such huge gaps in how we evolved back then and how we live today, it isn't hard to understand why we modern humans tend toward obesity and chronic disease with age. The current state of health in the world is a clear reflection of the incongruence of our genetic design as expressed in modern lifestyles. Our own country tells the most shocking tale, in spite of the United States being one of the wealthiest nations in the world—a fact that might lead you to expect it might be one of the healthiest, too. But we have the highest rates of obesity, more than any other country in the world.

In fact, health problems and chronic illnesses resulting from a diet of highly processed foods and a sedentary lifestyle pose a serious threat to public health. Over 66 percent of U.S. adults are overweight or obese, and 34 percent are obese. Obesity is estimated to cause more than 112,000 deaths per year. In addition, 64 million Americans adults have cardiovascular disease, 50 million have high blood pressure, and 11 million have type 2 diabetes. At least 7.2 percent of postmenopausal women develop osteoporosis, and 39.6 percent have osteopenia, a precondition to osteoporosis. Cancer is the second leading cause of death after cardiovascular disease, and it is estimated to cause 25 percent of all deaths in the United States.

All this disease exists despite the remarkable technological and pharmacological advances of the twenty-first century. Could the problem be that we are socially adapted to the twenty-first century but physiologically adapted to the Stone Age era? The solution in that case, I came to believe, was to align our lives with the lifestyle patterns of our Paleolithic ancestors—to move and eat as they did—which was the basis for Primal fitness theory and how I apply it in the Primal Body Program, described in Part 2.

DISCOVERING PALEO EXERCISE: ART DE VANY

After completing my degree, I kept up my interest and exploration in evolutionary fitness and discovered the work of Dr. Art De Vany, another Primal fitness theorist. At the time, De Vany was a professor of economics and behavioral sciences at the University of California at Irvine. He was also an accomplished athlete, with a background ranging from Olympic weight lifting to professional baseball; at age seventy-three, 6'1" and weighing 202 pounds, he measured 6.7 percent body fat, an impressive profile for a man his age, or any age.

Whereas Cordain had stressed diet in his research, only touching briefly on exercise and movement, De Vany synthesized a holistic approach to health and fitness that included both diet and exercise. Evolutionary Fitness, as he called his theory and also titled his seminal essay presenting his ideas, is based on the premise that our genes have encoded both behaviors and human physiology from a hunter-gatherer body and mind.

I had already been mimicking the early hunter-gatherer diet by adhering to a low-carb, high-protein, and healthy fats regimen, getting results not only for myself but for my clients as I advised them on their fitness goals. But I was curious about the exercise component of our ancestors' early lives. I knew that an active lifestyle was what made people healthy and that having more muscle and less fat on our body was congruent with our genes. But De Vany gave me an important piece that made it all come together—and coincidentally, paralleled the kind of training I had naturally found to be the most effective for weight loss, fitness, and health.

De Vany suggests that "our genes were forged in an environment where activity was mandatory—you were active or you starved or were eaten . . . diabetes, Alzheimer's disease, insulin resistance, heart disease and a whole modern panoply of chronic, long-lasting diseases are the product of genes that require activity for healthful expression." His idea is that exercise should mimic the activities of our ancestral past and "the key is to hit the right balance of intensity and variety . . . [because] intensity is the key to reaching the fast twitch fibers of the muscles, which are the key fibers to staying young."

This is very different from the physical activity recommendations made by most health professionals over the last four decades. Low-intensity, aerobic activity—not high-intensity activity, the kind that uses the fast twitch muscle fibers—is most often prescribed for fat loss, because it is believed that you burn more fat at the lower intensities. But the low-intensity approach is very shortsighted, because you only burn more fat during the time period you are exercising at the lower intensities. You burn more *total* fat when you exercise at higher intensities, due to what is known as the "afterburn effect," which causes you to continue to burn fat for up to 38 hours after exercise. (I explore this phenomena in more detail in Chapter 2 and show you how to put it to work for fat loss in Part 2, "The 5-Step Primal Body Program.")

At the time I discovered De Vany's approach, I had moved in my own training program from a focus on body-building exercises—isolation and compound movements to build muscle—to a focus on high-intensity intervals and functional strength training—a shift that required a different kind of movement. High-intensity interval training (HIIT) consists of short, rapid bursts of activity alternating with brief periods of rest. It is proven by study after study as the most effective form of cardiovascular exercise for fitness and fat loss, over the long term, which is why it is the backbone of the recommended exercises in the Primal Body Program.

De Vany's theory confirmed I was on the right track, when he described how early humans moved. They often sprinted, using short, intense bursts of speed, and then rested—the kind of pattern you'd expect for people who roamed the savannas in search of game. Also, our ancestors needed the cardiovascular power to be able to move quickly when predators threatened them—even more than the capacity for moving at moderate speeds over long distances. They needed to perform more explosive movement over short distances. Leaping and jumping were more likely physical skills that evolved, given the circumstances.

A fitness program modeled on our early ancestors' activities was exactly what I had been developing on my own. My program was composed of high-intensity sprints, functional strength training without machines, and a smaller amount of low-intensity "play" activities, such as running or hiking. What made my exercise program unique was the emphasis I placed on HIIT and the Primal movement patterns used in my functional strength-training component. Long-distance aerobic activities, such as running and hiking, complemented rather than dominated it.

No wonder it was working! A light bulb went on when I realized I had naturally evolved in my own routine to both eat and move as the earliest humans did. It explained perfectly the terrific results I had been seeing in myself and for my clients.

This was to make even further sense when I began training with kettlebells, those ball-shaped weights of varying sizes that are showing up in gyms everywhere.

One way we modern humans can mimic the high-intensity movements
humans is by working out with kettlebells. Such exercises as the swing ;
snatch cause your body to hit the kind of metabolic peaks that our ancest
perienced every day of their lives.

An added benefit of these ballistic movements is that through practicing total
body tension and relaxation while generating power from the hips, the muscles
of the pelvic floor get stronger. Stronger pelvic floor muscles lead to an improved
libido and enhanced sexual vitality. In Chapter 3, I will tell you more about how
Primal movement and exercise, such as working out with kettlebells, can increase
longevity and sexual health.

MODERN-DAY OBSERVATION: WESTON PRICE

A third part in my understanding of Primal fitness theory came through a man
named Dr. Weston Price. Price, a dentist and nutritionist living in the early 1900s,
was one of the earliest pioneers in doing the research that formed the basis for
Primal fitness theory. But unlike Cordain and De Vany, Price did his research on
humans still living the Stone Age lifestyle in his time.

As a dentist, Price noticed that the children of his patients were having dental
problems that their parents did not have. In particular, he observed a pattern of
crowded, crooked, or missing teeth and malformed dental arches. Price compared
this pattern with the beautiful teeth and excellent health of primitive cultures and
questioned whether our modern diet might be a reason for this difference.

In the 1920s, when distant areas of the globe were becoming accessible through
air travel, numerous primitive societies were still living as they had been for many
thousands, even millions, of years. This was a great time to compare the effects of
the modern diet to the primitive ancestral diet. Price recognized this opportunity,
and he and his wife spent ten years traveling over 100,000 miles, studying the nutritional health of numerous primitive societies.

Price observed that people in native societies had all thirty-two of their teeth,
perfectly fitting dental arches, and perfectly formed teeth, suffering little or no decay. But when modern foods became integrated into their primitive diet, he noticed
first dental decay and then the emergence of disease, in addition to the beginning
of crooked, malformed teeth and dental arches.

Analyzing samples of native and modern foods in the laboratory, Price determined that native diets contained more than ten times the vitamins and minerals

of modern foods. In particular, his analysis revealed that levels of the fat-soluble, animal-source vitamins A and D were significantly higher in native foods, when compared to modern processed foods. He also noted that the common factors among the native diets that accounted for superior health were an abundance of animal foods and fat nutrients. From this exploration, it became clear that primitive societies were not afflicted with any of the diseases that were plaguing Western civilization.

Price's book *Nutrition and Physical Degeneration,* published in 1939, described what he discovered as he traveled to the remote corners of the world, looking for answers to health and disease. Today, the Weston A. Price Foundation, which can be found online at www.westonaprice.org, is a nonprofit organization that shares the research of Dr. Price and is dedicated to restoring nutrient-dense foods to the American diet, through education, research, and activism.

CHALLENGES TO THE THEORY

As I continued to develop my 5-Step Primal Body Program, I encountered some opposition to the basic tenets of the theory. I want to include those arguments here—and my answer to them—for anyone who may likewise have questions about the basis of the Paleo lifestyle.[2]

Challenge number one: "The reason hunter-gatherers did not get the diseases of civilization was because most degenerative diseases are age-related, and because hunter-gatherers had shorter life spans, they would be less likely to manifest these diseases."

Reality check: It is true that the diseases of civilization most often produce mortality later in life, but the first signs of the disease usually begin much earlier. For this reason alone, comparisons between members of modern industrial and primitive societies in the same age group are valid. Indicators such as obesity, rising blood pressure, atherosclerosis, and insulin resistance are more common in modern humans, when compared to more primitive societies. Measurements of muscular strength and aerobic power are more common in primitive groups, when compared to members of modern day societies.

In addition, it is estimated that about 20 percent of hunter-gatherers we can observe in remote tribes today reach age sixty or beyond, and of these elder hunter-gatherers, almost all are completely free of any signs of disease. This evidence suggests that it is modern industrial life, which is so out of sync with the lifestyle for which our genome was originally selected, that causes what we have come to know as the diseases of civilization.

Challenge number two: "Human adaptability, the premise that humans are among the most adaptable mammals, able to adjust to many changing conditions, so are quite capable of adapting to modern industrial life and thriving. Other factors, then, would have to account for the current state of ill health and disease so prevalent in our society today."

Reality check: No doubt, our capacity for adaptability has allowed our species to survive and multiply in a variety of different environments, but this does not mean that our biology operates perfectly in all of these environments. As I've mentioned, a general biological rule specifies that organisms are the healthiest when their environment most closely resembles the conditions for which their genes were selected. Our adaptive capabilities may allow us to tolerate conditions short term with no immediate consequences to our health, but those short-term sacrifices are going to affect our health somewhere down the line. Given that our genes are coded for hunter-gatherer nutrition and activity patterns, the diseases of civilization may be the long-term consequence.

THE REAL EVIDENCE

While there are probably other objections and arguments to the theory, the results speak for themselves. Not only have I reaped the benefits of this lifestyle, I've been able to share this program with hundreds of clients who share my enthusiasm and conviction that the Primal Body Program is life changing, even life saving!

Today, I can truly say I am lean, fit, and pain free—absolutely pain free—as a result of following the Primal Body Program. I've been lifting heavy weights for twenty years. When I meet up with old friends from the hard-core gym where I used to lift, they ask me, "Don't your knees bother you? Aren't you having back problems?" My answer is no, because I'm in better shape now than I was back then.

Because my diet and exercise patterns are fully congruent with my DNA, I don't have the chronic inflammation in my body that most people have. Following the Primal Body Program has kept me in excellent shape and steadily carrying only 15 percent body fat over the years.

Don't just take it from me:

Alan's Transformation: A Complete Lifestyle Overhaul

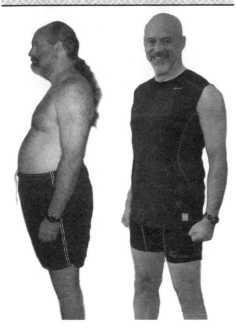

My client ALAN, a 54-year old computer engineer, shares how he transformed his body and lifestyle, using the Primal Body Program:

When I first started working with Mikki, I knew I needed a total lifestyle change. I had some health issues, like high blood pressure and back pain, and I was overweight—266 pounds. I'd been leading a pretty sedentary, fast-food kind of lifestyle for about 30 years, and always knew that when I reached a certain age, all that was going to have to change.

I got especially motivated after opening the newspaper one day and seeing the USDA's latest charts on height and weight. According to them, I fit into the category of "morbidly obese." I thought about doing the liquid diet, but I decided against it, because I didn't want something short term and extreme; I wanted a lifestyle change. I went to Weight Watchers and lost 40 pounds but soon hit a plateau and knew getting down any further was going to

require some kind of exercise program. That's what got me to the gym, where I met Mikki and started working with her as my personal coach.

My first workout sessions were intense. When I started, I couldn't even stand on one foot for an extended period of time. Some things Mikki had me do seemed bizarre, really wacky! She had me kneel on an exercise ball and balance while lifting weights, a routine that called on all my muscles to work together—but I could barely do it. But I pushed on until I started "bonking," a term used to explain the strange visual effects I was experiencing after an intense workout. This was due to low blood sugar and so I learned to drink a little juice after my session to provide some quickly digestible sugars. When I started changing my diet more toward the Primal diet, I noticed the bonking stopped happening.

When Mikki approached me with the idea of the Primal diet—high protein, healthy fats, and low carb—I was ready to hear it, even though I may not have been initially convinced. Today, my diet is radically different. Breakfast is a chicken thigh or some other protein food that I can eat quick on my way out the door. Not the normal American breakfast! But I find it to be very satisfying, and it starts me off well for any physical activity during the day. And of course, my weight is down in the range where I want it to be, which at my height of 6' 0" is 186 pounds.

I recently found I have a minor heart problem, which didn't surprise me since there's a history of heart problems in my family. I take a beta-blocker to manage it, but the last time I went in for an exam, my doctor was apologetic that there was nothing wrong—my blood pressure was right in range. I know this is a result of my Primal diet, and also the elimination of salt. I'm active now and keep in shape by working out, which helps, too.

I've come a long way. I started out doing step-ups, using a box that was 11 to 13 inches high. It was easy enough to step up on the box, but walking up and down stadium steps is something I couldn't do—ten would exhaust me. Now, I'm able to run the steps—twelve full stadium stair intervals (eighty-four steps each) in 15 minutes! The afterburn effect kicks in, and I burn calories like crazy. Another high-intensity exercise I learned to do was to leap sideways over an obstacle, and then go back and forth multiple times. Again, the afterburn effect kicked in for added burn.

I think of my progress as happening in stages, each stage marked by my being ready to hear something new, to try what might have seemed crazy but actually worked incredibly well. The improvement I've seen is astounding. My body fat percentage is 10.2 percent, and I'm stronger than I've ever been in my life—I can deadlift 245 pounds. My coordination, balance, and stamina are all greater than ever, and the back pain I used to have is completely gone.

NEXT . . .

Primal fitness works for weight loss, as well as health, longevity, and freedom from pain. In the next chapter, I will explain exactly how you can use this program to attain your weight-loss goals, including the story of my client who lost 100 pounds by following the Primal Body Program.

Chapter 2

Losing Weight
the Primal Way

Our caveman and cavewoman ancestors never had an issue with obesity or weight loss. The scientific evidence tells us they had an exceptionally lean and muscular body, as contrasted to modern humans who average 25 percent body fat for men and 35 percent for women. There are the obvious explanations for our ancestors' trim condition: periodic scarcity of food and a physically active lifestyle. But the story of how early humans naturally stayed lean, fit, and healthy only begins there.

In this chapter, you will learn how our ancestors' food choices carved the human genome for millions of years to turn their bodies into healthy, highly efficient fat-burning machines. I will show you how you can mimic their diet and use their genetic adaptation to achieve your weight-loss and fitness goals. When you mimic your ancestors' diet, you fully express your genetic inheritance, tapping into the ancient DNA that still keeps your body functioning as a healthy modern human being.

GENES AND YOUR DIET

Scientists give us plenty of evidence that mimicking our ancestors' diet is the best way to be healthy and lean, based on studies of the human genome. Since the Human Genome Project was completed in 2003, approximately twenty-five thousand genes have been identified in the human body, and a wealth of information has become available about how nutrition impacts our genes at the cellular level to create health or disease. The growing science of nutrigenomics, a new discipline that studies the relationship between nutrition, genetics, and health, is a direct result of this project. Nutrigenomics is based on the simple premise that dietary chemicals affect the expression of genes—for health, fat loss, and longevity.

Here's how it works: Most of the time, when you eat a meal, your body metabolizes the food to provide a usable form of energy for the cell, adenosine triphosphate, referred to by the acronym ATP. But sometimes dietary chemicals don't get metabolized to provide energy as ATP; instead they become ligands, or messenger molecules, that attach to proteins and "turn on" certain genes. These genes can either move you toward chronic illness or restore your body to health, making what you eat a potentially powerful influence on your physiology.

In her book *Primal Body, Primal Mind*, Nora Gedgaudas reports that "even by the most conservative standards in genetics, we actually control anywhere from a 'low' of 80 percent to upwards of 97 percent or more of our own genetic expression with respect to potential disease processes, and even longevity. Genes are turned on and off by regulatory genes, and regulatory genes are controlled mainly by nutrients. . . . There is no drug anywhere that can regulate genetic expression better or more powerfully than diet."

There are many examples of how diet and genes have evolved together. When our ancestors migrated out of sub-Saharan Africa sixty-five thousand years ago and began to populate southern Asia, China, Java, and later Europe, they met varying environmental conditions. Subgroups that formed on different continents around the globe adapted to these different dietary and environmental conditions, creating certain gene variants.

For example, if your earliest ancestors are from northern Europe, you can probably digest milk products with little difficulty. In most humans, a gene for lactose tolerance switches off once a person is weaned from mothers' milk, making it difficult to digest milk products. But a mutation occurred in the DNA of an isolated population of northern Europeans about ten thousand years ago, creating an adaptive tolerance for milk. As a result, descendants from this region can tolerate dairy today, whereas those who evolved in Asian regions cannot.

Of course, most of our genes are very old and evolved over the long period of time when we lived as hunter-gatherers. Studies by geneticists reveal that the DNA of all modern humans can be traced to a single female ancestor who lived in Africa about 140,000 years ago and a male ancestor who also lived in Africa 60,000 years ago. (However, this doesn't mean that male and female were the first modern humans; rather, it indicates that only their descendants survive to the present day, all others having fallen by the evolutionary wayside and not having made it to present time.)

Today, the human genome still contains many genetic traits of our earliest human ancestors and their contemporaries, so a healthy human diet would mimic the diet of ancestral humans. Although we recognize that there has been some genetic diversity and adaptations to different environments, it is scientifically sound to begin with the diet of ancestral humans because of our evolutionary history.

FOOD, HORMONES, AND FAT

As we have seen in Chapter 1, our ancestors ate a diet of mainly animal protein and fats with some carbohydrates, consisting of nonstarchy, fibrous plant food they pulled from the ground or plucked from a bush. They ate none of the foods we classify as carbohydrates today: starches and sugars found in grains, rice, potatoes; sugar, natural and industrial sweeteners, such as high fructose corn syrup; and fruits and sugar in dairy products. Theirs was naturally a low-carb, high-protein, and high-fat diet that kept their body functioning optimally for more than forty thousand years.

Our ancestors' diet is the basis of the Primal Body diet I recommend for you to keep your modern body lean and healthy. A key is how our food interacts with an important hormone, insulin.

Contrary to what many diet gurus have advised, excess body fat comes from eating carbohydrates that are converted into fat by the action of insulin. Most overweight people became overweight because of a condition known as hyper-insulinemia, or elevated insulin levels in the blood. This is a problem our ancestors didn't have to deal with, because they ate so few carbohydrates, their levels of glucose and thus insulin were low. Elevated insulin didn't make them fat, but it does make modern humans fat.

Let's take a look at how a diet typically high in carbohydrates and low in protein and fat—the exact opposite of our ancestors' diet throughout most of our evolutionary history—can lead to elevated levels of insulin and cause the alarming rates of obesity so prevalent in our modern lives.

Insulin has been with us over evolutionary time, carrying vital information to control the amount of sugar, or glucose, circulating around in your blood. When glucose is high due to eating a lot of carbohydrate foods, insulin from the pancreas is poured into the blood to help cells open their little doors (receptors) and admit the glucose. The cells need glucose as vital nourishment to run many important bodily functions—for example, using your brain to think and be able to read the words on this page.

You've probably heard of insulin in connection with diabetes, a disease that occurs when insulin fails in its job to control blood sugar levels and damage to organs results. What you may not know is that insulin has another job, one that was of importance to our ancestors, which is to store fat and other nutrients away in cells to be used later in times of famine—a condition that occurred often during

Paleolithic times. In its role to store away nutrients, insulin ensures that sugar is stored as glucose in the muscles and liver; amino acids, the building blocks of protein, are moved into muscle cells; and fat is stored away in fat cells.

All of the regulating activity occurs in response to what you eat. When you eat carbohydrates found in starches (grains and beans) and sugar (fruit and sweeteners), a metabolic signal is sent out to raise levels of insulin to store glucose in the muscles and liver. Eating protein from meat, fish, poultry, and eggs sends a metabolic signal to raise levels of both insulin, the fat-storage hormone, and also glucagon, a fat-mobilizing hormone that opposes insulin.[1] The rise in insulin drives amino acids into the cells so that the body can use them to build muscle. The rise in glucagon signals the body to release stored fat, so that it can be burned for fuel. Fats and oils found in meats, poultry, fish, butter, coconut oil, lard, olive oil, avocados, and nuts send a neutral signal, stimulating the release of insulin, but to a much lesser degree than carbohydrate or protein does.

When you follow the ancestral diet and eat mostly fibrous carbohydrates from vegetables and greens with little sugar or starch content, you will easily maintain blood glucose levels within the optimal range of 70 to 90 mg/dl. Your body is extremely meticulous about maintaining this range, because excess sugar circulating in the blood can be damaging to blood vessels, organs, and tissues in the body.

Here is an example of how your body is genetically designed to function best on a low-carb, high-protein, and high-fat diet: There are many hormones whose job it is to raise glucose levels for quick energy in an emergency situation—epinephrine, norepinephrine, cortisone, and growth hormone. These quick-energy hormones were a necessary adaptation so our hunter-gatherer ancestors could make a quick getaway from predators. But only one hormone evolved to lower glucose—insulin. Why? Because in evolutionary time, the human body has had little need to keep blood sugar lowered due to low carbohydrate intake.

In sum, our body was not genetically designed to have insulin play such a dominant role in regulating energy. Our modern diet makes insulin work overtime, and we pay a price—because early humans didn't need to lower blood sugar, as carbohydrates were a rare, almost nonexistent addition to their diet.

THE PRICE WE PAY

With the onset of civilization and a shift to an agricultural way of life, the human body was challenged to adapt to a new diet and metabolize large quantities of sugar and starch. With that change came corresponding high levels of insulin, the hormone responsible for regulating glucose and storing fat—and the high price that chronically elevated insulin levels extracts from our body.

The first price you pay has to do with how your body stores fat. The average person can only store 300 to 400 grams of glucose in the muscles and 60 to 90 grams of glucose in the liver. When the liver and muscles are full of glucose, excess is converted in the liver to fat (triglycerides) and stored in fatty or adipose tissue. In other words, when you overeat carbohydrates—starches and sugars—you cause your body to automatically store fat.

Even worse, as insulin levels soar due to eating too much bread, pasta, grains, and pastries, that stored fat becomes "locked in," making it impossible for you to use your own stored body fat for energy. Not only is the excess starch and sugar stored as fat, but once stored, that fat remains in your cells, making you *stay* fat!

A second price you pay is how your health is affected by a diet high in carbohydrates. Those soaring insulin levels can reduce the ability of your cells to receive insulin's message, which is to open the door and admit circulating blood sugar. When cell doors are closed, glucose stays circulating in your blood, signaling the pancreas to send out more insulin. But when the backup insulin arrives and knocks on the cell door, there is no response, because the cell's receptor has lost all sensitivity. This loss of sensitivity is known as insulin resistance, and it begins a vicious cycle that creates high levels of insulin, an exhausted pancreas, and high blood sugar—a complex of events that heralds an early stage of type 2 diabetes.

Eventually, your exhausted pancreas can no longer keep up with the demand placed on it for insulin, and you develop full-blown diabetes. First, your liver cells lose their sensitivity to insulin. Eventually, other tissues lose sensitivity, until finally your fat cells lose sensitivity. Then, with all doors closed, there is nowhere left for blood sugar to go, and it starts to build up dangerously in your blood. This can lead to a host of new health problems. Surges of excess glucose and insulin can damage nerve and brain cells, blood vessels can become constricted, vision and kidneys can become damaged, and ultimately you end up on dialysis, need a limb amputated, or have a heart attack.

As you can see, maintaining insulin sensitivity—the ability of cells to admit glucose from the blood—is a highly desirable state in terms of both fat loss *and* health. When your cellular receptors are sensitive, you require very little insulin in your blood to signal opening. The lower the insulin is in your blood, the lower your risk for many of the diseases of civilization.

USE YOUR GENETIC ADVANTAGE

In terms of weight loss, when insulin levels are low, fat storage is nonexistent, and you can easily unload fat from adipose tissue where it was stored. This is how your body was designed to keep fat from accumulating, and you want to use this genetic advantage for optimal weight loss. You do this naturally when you combine the Primal Body diet, which is low in carbohydrates and high in protein and fat, with the right exercise program, as you will see in Part 2 of this book.

In addition to eating a diet low in starches and sugars, adding more protein to your diet can help you tap into your body's genetic blueprint to lose weight and stay healthy. When you eat sufficient protein—grass-fed beef, free-range poultry, wild fish—stored fat is mobilized by the hormone glucagon. Glucagon helps move fat out of storage, so it is no longer locked in your cells, and it becomes available to be burned as fuel.

Bottom line, when you eat the way our ancestors did, the way we evolved to metabolize our food over eons of time, you cause your hormones—insulin and glucagon—to work for you to burn fat, stay lean, and keep excess weight off. With a diet low in carbohydrates—sugar, grains, starchy vegetables—insulin levels stay low to eliminate fat getting locked away and unavailable for use as fuel. Then, insulin resistance that causes disease and increased fat storage does not develop, because glucose is easily taken up by your cells as fuel.

ONE OF THE SECRETS TO BURNING FAT

Avoiding fat storage through limiting carbohydrates in the diet is helpful for weight loss, but if you want to burn fat, you have to do more than lower your insulin levels. To get your body to burn fat efficiently, you must create a need for fat as fuel. If you are already eating enough food to meet all of your energy requirements, your body has no need to call up its fat reserves. Cellular doors may be open, but fat not needed for fuel stays inside.

To lose weight, you must create a caloric deficit, which is a shortage of calories from food. A caloric deficit gets your body burning its own fat reserves for energy, an optimal situation for weight loss. How do you create a caloric deficit? First, figure your maintenance level of calories from food and then eat to drop down below it. Combining the resulting calorie deficit with a low-carb, high-protein diet will turn your body into a fat-burning machine. (In Chapter 9, I will show you how to create your own individual caloric deficit.)

METABOLIC ADDED EDGE

Another way you can get your body to burn fat is to take advantage of a little-known metabolic process our ancestors had going for them. Remember, your body is fussy about maintaining blood glucose levels within a narrow range and will work to insure adequate levels are maintained. On the low-carb Primal Body diet, you can lower your carbs to a level where your body has to manufacture glucose from protein to maintain optimal levels in the blood. This is done through a process known as gluconeogenesis—literally, making glucose from protein.

Gluconeogenesis requires many reactions in the body that consume and dissipate energy, burning an extra 200 to 300 calories in the process. This gives you a metabolic advantage by boosting your fat burning capacity. Our ancestors had this metabolic advantage working for them to burn fat naturally, because they ate so few carbohydrates.

Gluconeogenesis is one more reason why ancestral bodies were efficient fat-burning machines, and why yours can be, too. From our discussion, it's clear that a calorie is not a calorie. Why? Because a diet that is lower in carbohydrate but higher in protein and fat causes more weight loss than does a diet that is largely carbohydrate, even if caloric intake is the same.

KETONES: FAT-BURNING ALTERNATE FUEL

We know that our hunter-gatherer ancestors did not have abundant sources of carbohydrates in their diet, as we do today, and therefore had low levels of glucose circulating in their blood. In fact, there were times when they would go for weeks at a time with no food at all, so no glucose was on hand to nourish brain and tissues for vital functioning. During such periods of fasting/starvation, the challenge to the metabolism of early humans was to provide enough glucose, so they could continue to function until food was found.

As I have explained, glucose is in part produced through gluconeogenesis, the process of converting protein to glucose, and enabled early humans to survive times of starvation. But this process came at a price, because the protein needed to produce glucose is human muscle. Using precious muscle to make glucose could never be a long-lasting solution for our ancestors, because muscle was needed to hunt and gather food to survive and, therefore, couldn't be depleted without threatening their very survival.

An evolutionary adaptation was the creation of another source of internal fuel: ketones. Ketones are a by-product of gluconeogenesis, created when the liver burns fat to convert protein to glucose. Contrary to what you may have heard, ketones are a safe and effective source of fuel. In fact, they are the preferred fuel for almost every organ and tissue in the body. By providing this additional source of fuel during times of starvation, ketones spared muscle, lessening the demand for bodily protein sources in converting glucose for fuel.

The point is that your muscle is a valuable reserve of protein that can be used for glucose production, when needed. But the body prevents too much loss of muscle over long periods of starvation by boosting its production of ketones, a process known as ketosis. In contrast to our ancestors, we modern humans are not starving from any lack of glucose and, therefore, don't need to worry about wasting muscle to get sufficient glucose—our diet gives us plenty. However, the evolutionary adaptation of ketosis can be useful for weight loss. When you eat a low-carb diet—just low enough so that your liver still has to convert some protein into glucose—you want to be sure you eat enough animal protein for conversion, so that your muscles aren't required in the process.

The amount of carbohydrate needed to reach the state of ketosis varies for each person, but generally fewer than 50 grams of carbohydrate per day will take you to a place where you can achieve a significant amount of fat loss while maintaining your lean body mass. This is a very effective approach to weight loss.

A key element of the Evolutionary Fitness approach to health is to keep glucose levels in the body low. Glucose alters gene expression in a profound way because it is a substance that was comparatively rare during the evolution of our genes. We who are part of the growing Evolutionary Fitness community know that glucose is an essential internal fuel. But we do not obtain it from external sources; we rely on the glucose that is produced internally through gluconeogenesis—a system the body controls closely to produce only the amount of glucose demanded by the brain.

—ART DE VANY (ARTHURDEVANY.COM)

Once you gain experience with your body's fat-burning state of ketosis, you can begin to regulate your body fat naturally without any great effort. It becomes almost instinctive. Why wouldn't it?—humans have been living on ketogenic diets for almost 3 million years!

HUNGER AND THE PRIMAL BODY DIET

Many of my clients are 30 to 40 pounds overweight when they first come to me. When I introduce them to the Primal Body diet, they often tell me that cutting carbs would be too difficult to maintain. "I'd be hungry all the time," they say. This is an understandable response, because almost everyone who is that much overweight has chronically elevated insulin levels, and therefore depends on the quick fix of eating carbs to quell hunger.

As I've mentioned, when your insulin levels are high, fat is locked away in your fat cells. This is a problem, because your body requires constant nourishment and is not getting it from the stored nutrient. To compensate, your body takes in extra nourishment (and calories) during meals and then locks it away in your fat cells, where it cannot be accessed when needed after the glucose in your blood is used up.

Once your cells have taken up all the glucose, your blood sugar drops and you feel hungry. Hunger occurs even though there is an abundance of nourishment stored in your fat cells. So you grab a sugary snack and get the response your body wants, and your blood sugar comes back up. But so does your insulin, causing more of the fat storing activity, making it less available and so requiring more food for energy. You're hungry again. This cycle goes on and on, taking you on a rollercoaster ride as blood sugar and insulin bounce up and down. It soon becomes a habitual response to unconsciously ply your body with carbs at every snack and meal, to manage the highs and lows. Calling it quits would mean you'd risk experiencing the mood swings that often accompany sustained drops in blood sugar. No wonder my clients who are overweight say cutting the carbs is just too difficult!

When you switch to a low-carb Primal Body diet and start eating more protein and fat, things begin to change. A meal consisting of roast leg of lamb with sautéed Swiss chard sends a completely different signal to your body than does pasta and a salad. The meat and vegetable meal provide protein and fat with a little carbohydrate, so your insulin levels are elevated minimally, and fat stores remain available as fuel.

Also, because you ate the animal protein, your glucagon (insulin's opposing hormone) levels go up, stimulating your body to mobilize the stored fat in your fat cells for energy. If you do require more glucose because your meal was low-carb, the leg of lamb provides an abundant source of protein for conversion (gluconeogenesis), granting you not only the extra glucose but the metabolic advantage from those calories expended in the process. As a result, your cells get the nourishment they need, and you feel sated and begin to lose that unwanted fat.

LEPTIN: NATURAL HUNGER CONTROL

As if lowering insulin levels and increasing fat mobilization weren't enough of a fat-burning benefit from the Primal Body diet, an additional adaptation gives another advantage—the hormone leptin. Remember, hormones are communicators, and leptin's job is to send a message to your brain to suppress appetite. But leptin's job is much bigger than that. Leptin essentially controls metabolism by regulating all of your body's energy stores; it is a master hormone that regulates your body's response to starvation.

It works this way: When your fat cells are full, they send a signal via leptin to the hypothalamus in your brain, essentially saying, "Hunting is good, food not needed." You cease to feel hungry. As time passes, your fat cells get smaller and produce less leptin, which sends a signal to your brain that you need more fuel. You then experience hunger and get ready to go out for the hunt—or take a trip to the nearest grocery store.

Why then, you may ask, if we have leptin regulating our hunger so regularly, is obesity such a problem? Why don't people who are overweight, with plenty of fat stored in their bodies, get the signal that hunting is good, and therefore curb their appetite? And even more puzzling, why do people with lots of fat on their body constantly complain that they are hungry?

The answer is this: Just as there is insulin resistance, there is also leptin resistance, and the same foods that trigger insulin resistance—starches and sugars—also disrupt leptin function. The reason is that carbohydrates cause an increase in triglycerides, which is fat circulating in the blood. When triglycerides are high, leptin is blocked from crossing over the blood brain barrier to reach the brain, and the brain doesn't receive the satiety signal to turn off the hunger. In short, leptin cannot do its job when you eat a high-carb diet.

Your Ice Age primal body and mind are ruled by leptin. Adequate, not excessive, dietary fat—in the absence of dietary carbohydrates—is the optimal key to unlocking its power and potential to controlling your health, your well-being and your life span.

—NORA GEDGAUDAS, *PRIMAL BODY, PRIMAL MIND*

How do you know if you have leptin resistance and are experiencing hunger when you are well nourished? Here are some of the symptoms, as reported in *Primal Body, Primal Mind* by Nora Gedgaudas:

- Being overweight
- Fatigue after meals
- The presence of "love handles"
- High blood pressure
- Constantly craving "comfort foods"
- Feeling consistently anxious and/or stressed out
- Feeling hungry all the time or at odd hours of the night
- Having osteoporosis
- Unable to lose weight or keep weight off
- Regularly craving sugar or stimulants (like caffeine)
- Having high fasting triglycerides over 100 mg/dl—particularly when equal to, or exceeding, cholesterol levels
- A tendency to snack after meals
- Problems falling or staying asleep
- Your body seems to look the same, no matter how much you exercise

The way to restore leptin function is to eat the low-carbohydrate diet our ancestors did, because when you eat less carbs, you reduce your triglyceride levels. When triglycerides are low, leptin can easily pass through the blood-brain barrier and deliver the message to the brain that fat cells are full—once again, hunting is good, food not needed. This is why it's so easy to stay on the low-carb diet once you get on it—there's no hunger and you feel satisfied after eating.

When I ask clients who did not expect to be able to stay on the low-carb diet how they feel after losing a significant amount of weight, most comment that they never feel hungry. They also are surprised at how good they feel and how easy it is to maintain the low-carb, high-protein lifestyle. Not only do they feel better, but they have more energy, and so feel more like being active and exercising. Movement becomes desirable, which was our ancestors' experience when they ate a similar diet.

By now, you can understand how the low-carb, high-protein, and high-fat diet of our hunter-gatherer ancestors kept them lean and muscular, turning their bodies into healthy and efficient fat-burning machines. There are many different pathways that your genetic code has evolved for this purpose, and if you bring your lifestyle choices congruent with your genes, you will have the foundation to build a lean, fit, and healthy body.

EFFORTLESS FAT LOSS: THE DYNAMIC WEIGHT STAGE

Whenever I tell my clients about the dynamic weight stage, they get very excited. Who wouldn't get excited to learn that your fat loss can gather so much momentum, it continues no matter what or how much you eat? Let me tell you my own experience with this phenomenon.

I've had a lot of practice with weight loss over the years, not because I've been overweight myself, but because I wanted to maximize my body composition for competitive presentation. In 1992, I dieted down to 6 percent body fat to compete in the Iron Maiden bodybuilding contest. In addition, I've helped many of my clients reach their ideal weight.

I've noticed that there's a point you can reach where you seem to have an incredible amount of momentum—whether you're gaining or losing. For example, when I was a couple of weeks out from my bodybuilding contest target date, I realized I had "peaked" in my weight loss and arrived at my goal too soon. So I tried to reverse course by eating more food, and found that no matter what I ate, I just kept losing.

You may be thinking you'd like to have that problem, and the fact is, you can. I've observed a similar phenomenon with some of my clients. One client in particular lost over 50 pounds, and when he finally reached his ideal weight, it seemed he could not slow down the fat-loss process. At first, he thought he might have some kind of wasting disease, such as cancer, but that was not the case. In a short time, he was once again able to reverse the trend and gain weight.

Dr. Michael Eades mentions this phenomenon, referring to the dynamic weight stage in his blog. Here's an excerpt from his blog:

> If you want to be successful . . . you've got to follow a low-carb diet . . .
> until you get to what was called in the old medical literature the "dynamic

weight stage" . . . when weight is changing rapidly in either an upward or downward direction. Anyone who has gained or lost a lot of weight has experienced this. . . . But you have to commit for a few solid weeks to get there. You can't . . . go on a few days and off, fill up on calorie-dense, low or no-carb junk, say you're doing a low-carb diet, and wonder why you aren't losing. You've got to get up into the low-carb saddle and ride.[2]

Eades makes the point that because of the dynamic weight stage, you want to be consistent in choosing low-carb foods and not veer from the diet. That way, you can build the momentum needed for what may seem like effortless fat loss. It's so much easier than starting and stopping over and over again and takes a commitment on your part to make it work.

PRIMAL EXERCISE TO BURN FAT

Eating low-carb, high-protein, and high-fats is one way to turn your body into an efficient fat-burning machine, but equally as important to reach your weight loss goal is the exercise and training program you choose.

As with diet, when we mimic the movement and activity patterns of early hunter-gatherers, we tap into a genetic blueprint that hasn't changed in forty thousand years. Human anatomy and physiology has remained relatively unchanged since our ancestors leaped from a cliff to escape a saber-toothed tiger or dragged a mammoth carcass over long distances back to camp. While today you probably aren't going to be fleeing predators or taking home animal kill, you can imitate those ancestral activities in how you exercise, taking advantage of your natural genetic ability to burn fat and stay fit and healthy.

Three evolutionary adaptations early humans made in response to their environment are key to the recommendations you will read about in Part 2, "The 5-Step Primal Body Program." The first is building muscle through functional movement, and the second is burning fat through high-intensity interval training, most effective when combined with resistance training. A third pattern of movement our ancestors engaged in is referred to as play, consisting of low-intensity aerobic activities, such as dancing, hiking, swimming, and other recreational kinds of movement.

In regard to strength or resistance training, it's well known that the more muscle you have on your body, the more fat you burn, because muscle is metabolically active tissue. Even at rest, muscle is burning energy, and the amount it burns is more than fat burns at rest. Quite simply, if you develop more muscle and have a higher muscle to fat ratio in body composition, you burn more energy and more stored fat as a result.

BODY COMPOSITION AND INSULIN SENSITIVITY

You've seen how a low-carb diet can keep you sensitive to insulin and thus avoid storing fat, but did you know that your body composition—whether lean and muscular or mostly fat with little muscle—affects insulin sensitivity, too?

In a recent study,[3] Loren Cordain and others wanted to understand the relationship between body composition and insulin resistance. The researchers noted that until about fifty years ago, proportions of muscle and fat on the modern body remained similar to ancestral ratios. They compared the physiques of preagricultural adults, based on skeletal remains, with those of modern elite athletes and determined that body compositions were similar—in both groups, males had about 10 percent body fat, and females had about 15. They then compared these statistics to average modern humans and found that males have greater than 25 percent body fat, while females have more than 35 percent.

Even more important, this evolutionary change in body composition can affect insulin circulating in your blood, and thus your health and fat-burning ability. (Remember, high levels of insulin are not desirable, creating a condition known as insulin resistance and decreasing the ability of your cells to take up glucose.) The mechanism is this: Because fat cells and muscle cells compete for circulating insulin, relative to your proportion of muscle to fat, your body composition determines how insulin is distributed when it is released from the pancreas. And since insulin receptors on muscle cells are much more efficient at glucose uptake than those on adipose (fatty) tissue, fitness level is a big predictor in glucose uptake. In other words, an individual in better condition with more muscle may induce seven to ten times more glucose uptake than may someone with more adipose tissue.

The point is that a lean, fit, muscular person will have much greater insulin sensitivity than will an out-of-shape, overweight person. Additionally, an imbalance of fatty tissue receptors relative to muscle cell receptors requires the pancreas to secrete extra insulin, which leads to insulin resistance. Bottom line, having more muscle on your body will improve insulin sensitivity, because muscle cells are more efficient at glucose uptake than are fat cells.

The rapid increase in insulin resistance seen by doctors in recent years occurred much too quickly to have been caused by changes in DNA. Rather, Loren Cordain and his team suggest that the increase is the result of the population's change in body composition. We have more fat on our body and therefore higher levels of insulin leading to resistance, obesity, and disease.

Winning the Battle of the Bulge: It's Not Just About Diet

Putting more muscle on your body improves insulin sensitivity, which is a good reason to lift weights and gain muscle. Better yet, you can combine strength training with intervals in metabolic resistance training (a strength-training session using a series of multijoint exercises with brief rests between sets). The reason metabolic resistance training is better than strength training alone is because high insulin sensitivity requires not just muscle, but muscle FITNESS. Muscle fitness is measured by the VO2 max (maximum volume of oxygen that can be utilized in one minute of exercise) of the muscle, and figures into the insulin efficacy equation in the following way:

$$\text{insulin efficacy} = \frac{\%\ \text{muscle mass} \times \text{VO2 max}}{\%\ \text{fat mass}}$$

If you do metabolic resistance training to build strength and conditioning, you improve your body composition, creating more muscle and less fat. But you also improve your glucose uptake, and as a result have less circulating insulin, so you store less fat. It's how to win the battle on obesity!

Anyone who tells you that exercise alone does not affect weight loss is clearly missing this point. It's not about how many calories you burn in response to exercise; it's about changing your body composition through strength training and improving the VO2 max of the muscle. This is the link; it's why exercise is so important in the obesity epidemic. IT'S NOT JUST ABOUT DIET.

But having extra muscle does not provide as much advantage for burning fat as was originally thought. The resting metabolic rate of muscle is only about 6 calories per pound, whereas fat burns about 2 calories per pound. The majority of your resting energy expenditure actually comes from the activities of your organs—kidneys, liver, heart, brain—which are just a small proportion of your overall body mass.

AFTERBURN IS KEY

The key to fat loss is something called exercise afterburn, which refers to the calories expended above resting values after you stop exercising.

Burn fat after you stop exercising? Yes, this is what our ancestors' bodies were so uniquely adapted to do, so when they engaged in high-intensity activities, their body continued to burn calories and fat, even while they rested sitting around the campfire, sometimes for days at a time!

Exercise scientists refer to the afterburn effect as excess postexercise oxygen consumption (EPOC). When you train for brief intervals at high intensities, your body goes into an "oxygen debt," such as when you quickly sprint up a hill and are caught short of breath at the top. This debt has to be paid back.

Furthermore, research suggests that the more muscle you have on your body, the more calories you burn *after* an intense workout. Chris Scott, PhD, exercise physiologist at University of Southern Maine Human Performance Laboratory, reports, "When exercise ends, it takes time and energy for muscle cells to return to resting levels. . . . Recovery can also be expensive: Depleted glucose and fat stores need to be refilled, accumulated cell products need to be removed, and protein levels need to be built back up. All this requires energy."

The amount of elevation in oxygen consumption and the duration of time that oxygen is elevated are two important factors in the afterburn equation. They in turn depend on two variables in your workout: how intense that workout is and how long it lasts—*intensity* and *duration*. The more intensely you work out over longer periods of time, the higher the elevation in oxygen consumption is and the longer that elevation lasts, extending afterburn benefits sometimes by a great margin. Generally, it takes anywhere from fifteen minutes to forty-eight hours for the body to fully recover back to a resting state.

How does this translate to the best kind of exercise you can do to burn fat most efficiently? As you will see in Part 2, in the 5-Step Primal Body Program, I recommend resistance (strength) training done along with high-intensity interval training, to take advantage of the afterburn effect. Several studies suggest that heavy resistance training elicits greater EPOC when compared to aerobic cycling, lower-intensity circuit training, and low-intensity aerobic exercise. An added benefit of resistance training is that you increase your muscle mass, and so progressively burn more calories following your workouts.

But high-intensity resistance training is not the only way to elicit EPOC. High-intensity interval training produces a significant afterburn as well. Studies have compared the effects of a continuous run (thirty minutes at 70 percent VO2 max) to an interval run (twenty bouts of one-minute duration at 105 percent VO2 max), and found significantly greater EPOC following the intermittent bouts of exercise.[4]

Fittingly, these patterns of movement and exercise parallel the movement patterns of our early ancestors who were required to use great strength (carrying that mammoth carcass) and also to respond in short bursts of intense speed (fleeing predators) to ensure their survival. It is no coincidence that what worked to keep them lean and fit will work for you!

Patty's Transformation: Losing Close to 100 Pounds

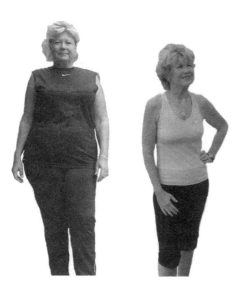

A former CEO, my client PATTY is now a strategic business coach and author. Here is her story of training with me and using the Primal approach to lose 100 pounds.

In the decade before I started the Primal Body Program, I'd allowed myself to get in very poor physical shape. Over the years, I steadily put on weight and finally topped out at around 260.

At 5' 10'' , that's a pretty large amount of weight to be carrying around.

Also, I was in a lot of pain. My feet were hurting so bad I could no longer wear high heels, and the arthritis in my knees was killing me. There were times when just sitting down in a chair was painful. I was taking aspirin every day, and I remember thinking to myself: I'M IN MY FIFTIES AND THIS IS NOT THE LIFE I INTENDED FOR MYSELF. I couldn't remain in denial much longer.

The turning point came while I was on vacation. I needed a bathing suit, so I went shopping to get one. Luckily, I found a Target that carried giant sizes, and I tried on a few suits in the dressing room. I remember looking in the mirror and feeling sick—it was a moment of truth.

I decided right then and there I would do something. I met Mikki and began working with her as my personal trainer. It's now been two years since I started the Primal Body Program—two years' and 100 pounds' difference!

I started working out twice a week and I learned to use a foam roller, a tool I've gotten a great deal of benefit from, especially for the pain in my knees. After I began to lose weight and get fitter, Mikki took me out to the college track, and we'd walk around it or run up and down the stadium stairs. In the first six months, I steadily dropped 8 to 10 pounds every month.

I also keep a food journal to stay on track with my new low-carb eating style, writing down all my food choices at each mealtime. Analyzing it, and with Mikki's coaching, I saw how I could choose to eat more animal protein—fish, chicken, or beef, for example—rather than automatically go for the potato or corn on the cob if I was still hungry. Slowly, bit by bit, I was able to change my eating habits, and now I eat protein and good fat at every meal, and take omega-3 fish oil capsules, along with other supplements.

The inflammation and pain in my joints started to go away. I was also taking the supplement glucosamine for my joints every day and doing a lot of work to strengthen the muscles around my knees, so I'd have less pressure on the arthritic parts. The combination of diet, supplements, and exercise made my knees get even better, and today, I don't have the arthritis pain any more. I can even wear high heels again! And I haven't had an aspirin in more than a year and a half.

On days I don't work out, I'll do something outdoors, like take a hike behind my house with the dogs. I never would have done that before because of the pain I was in, but now I work hard to plug exercise into my days. I naturally want to move my body and get sunshine, to debrief after a stressful day. And I know that this regular exercise is helping to keep my metabolism going strong, so my calorie-burning furnace is more efficient.

Most important, I feel like I have a valuable key to living a longer life with more energy and awareness. I have a much better ability to judge what's good for me and what's not. Recently, I was visiting my family and we went to a favorite eatery, the sort of very traditional, home-cookin' kind of restaurant, to have lunch. Ninety percent of the stuff they served there you wouldn't want to put in your body. Fried chicken, French fries, onion rings, and everything super sized. I thought, I USED TO EAT LIKE THIS ALL THE TIME. Luckily, I can go to a restaurant now and order a Cobb salad, knowing I'm doing something good for my body and my weight. I learned how to eat on the Primal Body Program, and that has stayed with me no matter where I go. The Primal Body Program is definitely an education—and it's such a fundamental shift in living, your whole life is affected by it.

NEXT . . .

In Chapter 3, you will learn what it takes to keep this program in your life, for the rest of your life, with an emphasis on healthy longevity.

Chapter 3

Live to Be 100 and Die Disease Free

What if you could live to be one hundred, and be pain and disease free, with all your mental faculties intact? If that were possible, would you want to extend your life and continue doing whatever you do that makes your life worth living?

Today, becoming a centenarian is more possible than ever before. The ranks of this elite club have swelled in the United States to 104,099 in 2009—up from 38,300 just twenty years ago. But being healthy and alert in later age is not usually how it goes. Most of us dread the thought of living to be one hundred, seeing the diseases of civilization claim friends and family members as they age. Even if you don't get cancer, diabetes, or cardiovascular disease, do you want to be one hundred years old with a body that can't move or think well?

Extended youthfulness, not merely prolonged life, is the goal, and modern science is pointing to exercise and diet as the key to reaching this fountain of youth. From what they are saying, a lifestyle that mimics our ancestors' and is congruent with our genetic inheritance is the ticket that will get us there.

PRIMAL LONGEVITY

James Fries, an emeritus professor at Stanford School of Medicine, coined the phrase *compression of morbidity.* By this, he meant you simply erase chronic illness and infirmity from the first 95 percent of your life. You live a healthy life year in and year out, until you expire from natural causes.

This, not decrepitude and painful decline, describes the lifeline of our hunter-gatherer ancestors, who lived a healthy life and died with plenty of muscle on their body. They may have met their end in the jaws of a saber-toothed tiger or drowned in a tar pit or bog, but as paleo-anthropologists have shown, the earliest humans didn't die of diabetes, heart disease, Alzheimer's, or cancer. So why should you?

Think about it: Animals in the wild don't die of debilitating old age, and we don't have to, either. The earliest remains show our ancestors rarely suffered the diseases we modern humans die from, largely due to our sedentary habits and high-carb, processed-food diets.

According to Art De Vany, modern aging is a kind of slow death: "What we call aging is really *sedentary aging* and *carbohydrate abuse*. The accumulation of damage [from these causes] over a longer time scale is what aging is in Western countries. . . . The aging [population] just die over a longer time scale than do acutely ill individuals."

In this chapter, I explore the latest science of longevity in light of what we now know about the lifestyles of our Paleolithic ancestors. The Primal Body Program lays the foundation for becoming a healthy, active human of any age, and building on that, I will show you how you can extend your youthful vitality by taking advantage of both dietary practices and exercise that ensure you live a long life with a fit and functioning body.

In the first part of this chapter, I show you how you can beat Mother Nature at her game by taking advantage of *caloric restriction* and *intermittent fasting*. In the second part of this chapter, you will learn of the latest, startling science that is showing how exercise affects both sexual vitality and longevity, with tons of evidence that "going Paleo" with the Primal Body Program is the best way to stay young and prolong youthfulness.

CALORIC RESTRICTION AND LONGEVITY

While mimicking ancestral lifestyles is the best way to create a lean, strong, and healthy body, it's important to remember that our genes evolved with one goal and one goal only: the ongoing reproduction of the human species. In other words, Mother Nature wants us to survive just long enough to reproduce, and then, once we have passed beyond our reproductive years, she loses interest in us. The design is not automatically supportive of healthy longevity. However, I agree with Nora Gedgaudas that we can beat Mother Nature at her own game by taking advantage of certain biological mechanisms that have evolved over time. The mechanisms are already there—we just need to know how to use them for modern-day longevity.

One of the ways you can beat Nature at her game is through caloric restriction, or the cutting-back of calories in your diet—simply said, eating less food. Science shows us in both animal and human studies, that caloric restriction contributes to longevity and health. As far back as the 1930s, researchers were studying caloric restriction in animals to see whether it might extend youth or slow down the aging process. They found that caloric restriction did indeed have the effect of improving health and extending life span in animals.

If there is a known single marker for life span, as they are finding in the centenarian and
laboratory animal studies, it is low insulin levels.
—RON ROSEDALE, MD (WWW.DIABETESHEALTH.COM)

Here are some of the benefits studies show can occur when calories are significantly cut back:

- Reduced DNA damage
- Enhanced DNA repair
- Reduced inflammation
- Reduced levels of cholesterol and triglycerides
- Reduced risk for developing diabetes
- Reduced body fat
- Immune system ages slower
- Lowered blood glucose and insulin
- Reduced buildup of plaques leading to Alzheimer's disease

To apply caloric restriction to humans, an approach called caloric restriction with optimal nutrition (CRON) has been suggested. This approach involves supplementing the calorie-restricted diet with added nutrition, because nutrient density is also a factor in increasing life span.

How does caloric restriction work to extend life in humans? Caloric restriction impacts genes in some beneficial ways. In studies of healthy subjects who have reached one hundred years or older, it's been shown that some lucky people activated a gene called sirtuins (SIRT-1)—the "longevity gene"—and as a result have enjoyed extended life, even though they have not lived a particularly healthy life. (This, however, is the exception and not the rule.) The SIRT-1 protein plays a key role in repairing DNA damage and so helps protect the integrity of the genome, which appears to be essential to longevity.

You may have heard of the recent discovery of a nutrient in red wine called resveratrol that stimulates the longevity gene. But the dosage required to get the benefit found in the studies would require the average person to drink one hundred glasses of wine for one dose! More recently, additional longevity genes SIRT-2 and SIRT-3, which play an important role in maintaining the health of the mitochondria, were discovered. Researchers have found that caloric restriction is the most powerful way to activate these life-extending genes.

INSULIN AND LONGER LIFE

While numerous studies have shown that caloric restriction is effective for slowing down the aging process, the underlying factor that makes caloric restriction so effective is the lowering of insulin levels.

Insulin is an ancient, single-celled molecule that has been around for millions of years. As you may recall from Chapter 2, insulin was at first thought to control blood sugar and store nutrients. But we now know that insulin's main role is in regulating life span by switching on and off genes responsible for repair and maintenance at a cellular level. For this reason, we can refer to insulin as "the aging hormone."

Insulin's role in aging was discovered in the 1990s, when researcher Cynthia Kenyon at the University of California was studying an ancient species of worm called *C. elegans*. Kenyon discovered a genetic mutation in the worm that had doubled the lowly creature's life span. This mutation, called the DAF-2 gene, basically encoded an insulin receptor on the worm's cells. In simple life forms, such as *C. elegans*, insulin has nothing to do with regulating blood sugar; its job is to regulate reproduction and life span. Further research has confirmed that insulin has the same effect of regulating reproduction and life span with all species, including humans.

Here's how insulin regulates life span: When insulin levels go down, genes are turned on that have the job of doing repair and maintenance of cellular damage. In evolutionary time, during times when food was scarce, this allowed humans to remain healthy long enough to survive and reproduce, by extending their lives during times of famine.

Remember, Nature is interested in us surviving to reproduce, so it makes sense that we are given a genetic advantage to survive times of no food. With repair and maintenance mechanisms in place at the cellular level—thanks to low insulin—we remain healthy until food becomes more available and we can finally reproduce. Therefore, when you keep insulin low by restricting calories, you are ensuring that your cells are kept in good repair and maintenance over time. In short, you can take advantage of this famine "loophole" to increase your longevity.

This understanding of how insulin is the "aging" hormone, should make you want to strive for low insulin levels to "turn on" genes that repair your cells and maintain their health, thereby enhancing your longevity. Following the Primal Body Program guidelines when making food choices is the best way to do this, because restricting what you eat keeps insulin low and impacts how long you live.

Restricting carbohydrates and sugar, it turns out, has even more of an impact on longevity than does restricting calories. In 2009, researchers from the University of Alabama examined the effect of dietary sugar consumption on healthy human lung cells and on lung cells that were precancerous. They found that restricting the consumption of sugar can extend the life of healthy lung cells and speed the death of precancerous ones. Again, genes were the key: Two key genes were affected by the decreased glucose in the cell: telomerase, which allows cells to divide forever, and p16, a gene that encodes an anticancer protein.

This research on glucose restriction, the onset of disease, and aging in humans supports the earlier findings on caloric restriction from animal studies done in the 1930s and suggests that human longevity can be achieved through reducing calories, especially carbs and sugars. "These results further verify the potential health benefits of controlling calorie intake," reported the principal investigator, Dr. Trygve Tollefsbol. "Our research indicates that calorie reduction extends the lifespan of healthy human cells and aids the body's natural ability to kill off cancer-forming cells."[1]

While there are many benefits to be had from caloric restriction—protection from disease and longevity being just two—I doubt that many people would voluntarily decrease their caloric intake by 30 to 40 percent and stay there for life. In my work with clients, I've seen people who wanted to lose weight resist creating a caloric deficit of just 250 to 500 calories to reach their goals. This is because some of the uncomfortable effects likely to be experienced when cutting back on calories by 30 to 40 percent include loss of energy, decreased mental focus, and loss of muscle. People get hungry, irritable, and depressed. Does this sound like the kind of life you would want to extend?

Fortunately, there is a gentler method for practicing caloric restriction that does not bring about such deleterious effects and is much easier to do than permanently cutting back the amount of calories you take in. This method is called intermittent fasting.

INTERMITTENT FASTING: THE EASY WAY TO GO

In years past, the practice of fasting was usually associated with religious or spiritual customs and traditions. Almost every major religion today includes some kind of dietary restriction as a spiritual practice: Christian Lent, Jewish Yom Kippur, and Muslim Ramadan. But now, a growing number of fitness enthusiasts are beginning to include intermittent fasts in their lives as a way to lose fat and improve overall health and longevity.

Intermittent fasting (IF) involves a period of fasting alternated with a period of eating. It makes perfect sense from an evolutionary point of view. Our Paleolithic ancestors went through regular cycles where food was either readily abundant or extremely scarce. Feast or famine was the environment our genes evolved in. Because of these cycles, we evolved with episodes of caloric restriction or deprivation.

As we have seen, during times of scarcity, genes responsible for repair and maintenance get turned on. These genes increase the production of key biochemicals, such as glutathione, which promote the repair of tissues that would not be repaired in times of surplus. It is this adaptation that allows cells to live longer.

Intermittent fasting can be done in a number of ways to alleviate the discomfort associated with long-term fasting. An alternate-day fast involves a feast day during which you eat all you want of the low-carb, high-protein diet for the entire day, and then fast the next day. You can continue this cycle of alternate-day fasting for as many days as you like. Another way to do intermittent fasting is to do a 24-hour fast once a week, once a month, or whenever you decide on a planned or unplanned schedule. Finally, you can skip a meal on a planned or unplanned basis and get the benefits of IF. For example, there is no need to eat breakfast every day, as skipping breakfast on a busy morning now and then may have the effect of repairing damaged cells. You could also skip dinner on that same day and eat only one meal for the day.

Scientists have explored IF as a way to stay healthy and benefit from caloric restriction. Researchers compared three groups of mice: those doing intermittent fasting (IF), those with nonintermittent caloric restriction (CR), and those allowed to eat at will or ad libitum (AL). The purpose was to measure the effect of intermittent fasting (alternate-day fasting) on various factors, such as how much the mice ate, and their body weight, fasting insulin, fasting glucose, and IGF-1 (an insulin-like growth factor). The scientists found that when mice were maintained on IF, their overall food intake did not decrease and their body weight was maintained. Nevertheless, intermittent fasting resulted in beneficial effects that met or exceeded those of caloric restriction, including reduced insulin levels and increased resistance of neurons in the brain to stress.[2] Intermittent fasting therefore has beneficial effects on glucose regulation and neuronal resistance to stress in these mice—effects that are independent of caloric intake.

What's interesting about this study is that even though the IF mice ate twice as much as the AL mice, while the mice eating a calorie-restricted diet maintained 40 percent less calories overall, the researchers found that the IF mice had lower glucose and insulin levels than the CR mice. It has been thought that some of the beneficial effects of caloric restriction are derived from the lowered blood glucose levels, because less sugar in the blood can lead to less glycation, or damage to proteins, and less oxidative damage. But in this study, you might wonder how the intermittent fasting mice could have had lower glucose and insulin levels, as they gorged on food whenever they had access to it, while the calorie-restricted mice were maintained on caloric restriction all the time.

In answering this question, the researchers suggest that by confining bouts of high-caloric intake to a limited-time window, such as in intermittent fasting, there are benefits that don't occur when meals are more frequent, as with the CR regimen. It is the alternating periods of eating and fasting (anabolism and catabolism), as in intermittent fasting, that trigger increases in cellular stress resistance and the repair of damaged cells induced by the fasted state.

These findings suggest that intermittent fasting can enhance health and cellular resistance to disease, even if the overall caloric intake is not decreased. Therefore, intermittent fasting is a better method than merely restricting calories, and is a lot more comfortable and doable by more people. This is a perfect example of how conforming to the way our body is genetically designed to work, keeps us young, eliminates disease, and even increases cellular stress resistance.

EXERCISE AND LONGEVITY

While what and when you eat plays a major part in your health and longevity, how you move and exercise may be even more important. Why? Because your genes are coded with the expectation of a certain level of physical exercise, based on the activities of our human ancestors. To give us an idea of their level of fitness, researchers suggest that preagricultural adults' body and muscles were similar to those of modern-day Olympic athletes!

One of the well-known consequences of aging for us modern humans is the loss of lean muscle mass. Scientists have examined whether healthy aging is associated with a particular genetic profile involving mitochondrial function and whether strength training could reverse this signature to that of younger men and women.

In this study, researchers took tissue samples of gene expression profiles from healthy older men and women who performed strength training two times a week for six months. The samples were taken both before and after the regimen, and then compared to tissue samples of younger men and women.

A gene expression profile measures how well an individual's mitochondria are working. You may recall that mitochondria are the energy furnaces of the cell that produce ATP. It has been suggested that mitochondrial dysfunction is related to loss of muscle and function in older adults. Mitochondrial function is measured by counting the number of mistakes the mitochondria makes when transcribing DNA to make such materials as proteins.

What is interesting about this study is that it was the first to examine the molecular "fingerprint" of aging in healthy, disease-free humans. The study found a complete reversal of the genetic fingerprint back to the levels seen in younger adults, as a result of strength training! The researchers said that the results strongly suggest that mitochondrial dysfunction is linked to aging in humans. But the good news is that strength training reverses aging! The researchers concluded that "following exercise training, the transcriptional signature of aging was markedly reversed back to that of younger levels for most genes that were affected by both age and exercise."

In the same study, the researchers also measured muscle strength. Before the exercise program, the older adults had 59 percent less strength than did the younger adults. But after strength training, the older adults improved by 50 percent; they were only 38 percent weaker than were the younger adults. The participants of this study worked out on a Universal Gym, performing machine exercises such as leg press, chest press, leg extension, leg flexion, shoulder press, lat pull-down seated row, calf raise, abdominal crunch, back extension, arm flexion, and arm extension. Imagine how much strength could have been gained had they used free-weight, functional exercises instead![3]

A ninety-one-year-old, record-breaking track and field star, Olga Kotelko who was featured in a *New York Times* article, is living proof of the effects of high-intensity training on aging. According to the editor of Masterstrack.com, Ken Stone, Kotelko threw a javelin more than 20 feet farther than did her closest age group competitor. She also ran 100 meters in 23.95 seconds, which was faster than the finalists in the eighty- to eighty-four-year category—two brackets down. Researchers biopsied the muscles of Kotelko to see whether they contained any mitochondrial defects that are the usual biomarkers of aging. Such defects cause angular muscle fibers to stop working, because they have become unplugged from the motor neurons that tell them to fire. The researchers reported that they didn't see a single fiber that had any evidence of mitochondrial decay.[4]

Exercise helps to prevent muscle from slipping away, but according to Mark Tarnopolsky, a professor of pediatrics and medicine at McMaster University in Canada, strength training in particular is the most effective. Pointing to a phenomenon known as gene shifting, he reports that strength training can activate a muscle stem cell that has a rejuvenation effect on the mitochondria. If Tarnopolsky is right, older adults who exercise can roll back the calendar. He has shown that after six months of strength exercise training done twice weekly, the physiological, biochemical, and genetic signature of older muscle is reversed nearly fifteen to twenty years.[5]

METABOLIC HEADROOM: AN AGING ADVANTAGE

We know that strength training reverses the effects of aging, but did you know that exercise also gives you an aging advantage known as metabolic headroom? This concept of exercise capacity was coined by Art De Vany and refers to the difference between *the most you can do* and *the least you can do*. De Vany points out that when the most and the least you can do are the same, then you are dead. This concept relates to aging in that often the difference between the most and the least decreases as you age. Maximizing the difference between the two, through exercise, would then increase longevity.

What kind of activities determine the most you can do and the least you can do? For the most, try the kind of exercise advised in Step 5 of my Primal Body Program, high-intensity intermittent training (HIIT), which provides maximal stimulus to the body. For the least, you would simply be resting with minimal stimulus. The difference between the two is what De Vany is calling metabolic headroom.

According to De Vany: "Adults lose about 5 per cent of their lean body mass per decade after they enter their thirties. Most of the muscle they lose is FT (fast twitch) fiber, because they cease . . . to live in the FT region. They settle into the ST (slow twitch) region, and, consequently, as they age their muscle fibers atrophy. . . . Their skeletons are vulnerable to falls, and their muscles are not strong or quick enough to keep them from falling, because their FT fibers atrophy. Keeping your FT fibers is the best way to stay young."

EXERCISE AND SEXUAL VITALITY

How does Primal fitness impact your sexual vitality, especially as you age? Many of my women clients of a certain age start out complaining of declining libido, but soon find their complaints disappear as they get fitter. That, along with my own personal experience and studies done on the subject, are pieces of the puzzle providing answers to the question of how exercise impacts sexual health—especially Primal fitness.

My own training involving kettlebells was the first clue. I had attended a three-day seminar with Pavel Tsatsoulinc, the Russian who trained the Special Forces in Russia and the United States, and who brought kettlebell training to the West. After years of advanced/heavy lifting, I discovered that, as a result of kettlebell training, I was getting in better shape. But an added benefit was that I noticed an increase in my sexual vitality right after completing the three-day seminar, and continuing as I adopted kettlebell exercises into my training routine.

The three-day training was intense. Prior to the workshop, I worked on the kettlebell snatch (an explosive overhead movement), so that I could pass the snatch test (one hundred snatches in five minutes), which was a requirement for the certification. Then, during the three-day workshop, we worked exclusively with kettlebells. By the end of each day, we had done literally hundreds of swings in addition to practicing the other kettlebell movements.

An explanation came when I read a report of a study done on women kettlebell practitioners, showing that many sexual benefits resulted after eight to twelve weeks of training. We all know that resistance training, in general (bench press, barbell row, barbell squat, etc.), increases testosterone levels, so libido usually increases when you lift weights. Also, developing a stronger core and more flexibility can lead to more athletic sex. But this study went further in explaining why swinging a cannonball with a handle was shown to lead to "higher levels of sexual arousal, much stronger and more easily attained orgasm, and even multiple orgasms for some women whom had not previously experienced them."

The key to why kettlebells are so great for women, I discovered, was the involvement of pelvic floor muscles (PFM) that are strengthened by the muscular contractions involved in swinging a kettlebell. According to Coach Stevo, an RKC instructor, "Stronger PFM contractions mean better blood flow through the PFM and then into and out of the clitoral erectile tissue before and after sexual arousal. This better blood flow may contribute to keeping androgens and other sex hormones circulating in tissue longer, thereby allowing further stimulation and continued orgasm."

Do we need any more motivation to use kettlebells in training to get fit? The science shows you'll benefit from an increased sex drive, increased ability to orgasm during intercourse, and an overall improvement in feelings of sexual satisfaction. Compare these benefits against the small amount of time necessary to strengthen the pelvic floor, and you'll agree with me that these exercises are something that should make their way into everyone's daily routine.

And not to exclude the guys, who can also benefit in sexual health from training with kettlebells: Pelvic floor muscle contraction works the prostate and increases blood flow to the penis, translating to a reduction in impotence, increased ejaculatory control, and increased orgasmic intensity. Good-bye, Viagra![6]

REVERSING AGING

In the past, aging has often meant a gradual loss of health and vigor as the years progress. We now know this slow decline is no longer inevitable. When you combine the right exercise and nutritional program with periods of intermittent fasting, even an unfit person can turn around most of the consequences of aging.

We know, for example, that VO2 max, the single best measure of cardiovascular fitness, decreases about 10 percent per decade once you've reached thirty years of age. Loss of lean body mass, another consequence once considered a natural part of the aging process, is now thought to result more from disuse and lack of exercise—sedentary living—rather than simply from getting older.

Adrienne's Transformation
Never Too Late

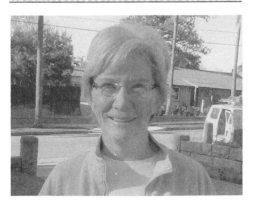

ADRIENNE is a seventy-four-year old retired career woman with two active grandchildren. In her own words, here's the story of her remarkable transformation.

I found Mikki through *C Magazine,* when she was written up as one of the top trainers in California. I signed up to train with her two times a week, and that was three and a half years ago.

At the time, I was a little overweight and prediabetic. I've always been very active, so I didn't have big weight problems. I'm 5'2" and at the most weighed 119. I didn't lose a whole lot of weight, but I did lose inches, and I'm so much stronger now than when I started.

One of my main reasons for getting in shape is to be able to care for and play with my grandchildren, to be up for that kind of activity. It's worked out beautifully. One of them weighs 37 pounds, and it's not a problem for me to lift her. Plus, my husband is younger than me, and I have to keep up with him. He's very athletic and sails competitively.

When I started the program, I couldn't do one roll-up—that was the condition of my midsection. I can do twenty-five now, and I'm that much older! It's not a big deal. I'm fitter too, more active, more healthy. I love working with 12-kilo kettlebells (26 pounds).

One of my really big successes with Mikki has been conquering sugar. It's made a huge difference in my life. I loved sweets, chocolate, candy—all desserts are wonderful, one of the great pleasures in life, and I was craving that stuff all the time. I still love it, but I don't crave it. I don't eat very much of it, because I don't want to get diabetes. My doctor was recommending drugs, but I told him I wanted to try a diet. He said a diet is going to take you a year. It probably did, but now I am no longer prediabetic and I did it without drugs.

I've also been tested for the Alzheimer's gene, and I do have it. My mother had it, and she deteriorated a lot around this age, but I get tested every six months and don't show any signs so far in deterioration. Mikki thinks the cut back in sugar in my diet makes it less likely that the gene will be turned on.

I keep a food diary intermittently, when I need to bring down my weight. We did it for a while to get me on track, but I'm very food conscious now. I went from eating a lot of sugar and a lot of carbs, to the point where I now eat Paleo style. For breakfast today, for example, I had eggs and ham and salad. Not the typical breakfast, and not what I was eating when I first started with Mikki—then, I was eating croissants!

At seventy-four, I set a new personal best recently, going up and down the stadium steps at our local school track. There are 840 steps, ten sets of 84 steps each. I did all of them, interval style, in a little less than thirty minutes. I thought it was amazing. It's like the roll-ups—I couldn't do steps at all when I started. We worked up to it slowly, and I think that's a key. It took a long time to get to this point. I'm not suggesting anyone my age go out there and sprint around if they're not used to it. You have to go slowly, which is why it's important to have a pro, somebody who can see what you're doing and guide you.

We've recently started setting short-term goals. I have goals now that are six-week goals, and Mikki keeps me on track for them. I set a goal, and she designs a program to meet that goal. I know for the next six weeks what I'm going to be doing. I ran a 5K this summer, and then I went on a 10-mile a day hike for a week through England. By the time I went, I knew I wouldn't have any trouble going for five days, at 10 miles a day.

My posture is better, too—I stand up straighter than I used to. I was rounded in my upper body, but since doing core exercises and strengthening the muscles in my upper back, I'm no longer that way.

So it's a success story at my age. . . .

The good news is that with the right type of exercise—strength training and high-intensity intervals—you can minimize or even reverse this trend. One of my clients reversed the aging process when she started exercising at age sixty, after a lifetime of never exercising. Adrienne started her training with me at the age seventy-one, and the story of her transformation is inspiring to anyone wanting to extend their life and live into a healthy old age.

NEXT . . .

You are now ready to be introduced to the five steps of the Primal Body Program, which follow in Part 2 of this book. The Primal Body Program is designed to maximize your body's ability to burn fat, so you can lose weight. Because health is also important, the program shows you how to achieve nutrient density with supplements that compares to the diets of our earliest ancestors, whose food was not depleted from modern industrial food practices, as is ours. Another focus is bringing down dangerous levels of inflammation that most of us have from our modern diet and sedentary lifestyles, giving you a chance to live an active, long, and healthy life. Finally, you will learn how to move in ways that are congruent with your genetic blueprint, so exercise is a natural extension of your day—something you *want* to do, not struggle to do.

As you follow the program, you can focus on one step or another, depending on your need and level, but all five steps need to be part of your program to get the best results. Sequence is also important, so even though you might favor one step over another, don't get ahead of your game; start with Step 1 and work your way through to Step 5. You'll be glad you did that by the time you arrive!

Remember, the Primal approach is a comprehensive shift, rather than a quick fix for a specific problem. While you may be addressing a specific problem such as weight loss, the design of the program calls for you to include all aspects of Primal fitness in achieving your goal.

PART II

The 5-Step
Primal Body Program

Chapter 4

Step One—Eat the Anti-Inflammation Primal Diet

STEP 1

The first step in restoring your body to the natural health and fitness of our Stone Age ancestors is to rid your body of what doctors have come to agree is the single greatest threat to our physical well-being: chronic inflammation. Since the late 1990s, study after study has come out showing chronic inflammation is involved in every disease of civilization, including cancer, diabetes, coronary heart disease, arthritis, Alzheimer's disease, autoimmune diseases, and even chronic fatigue syndrome.

Disease is certainly linked to inflammation, but joint pain is also caused by inflammation, a condition that stops people from getting exercise and keeps them sedentary. In Step 1 of the Primal Body Program, I will show you how to eliminate the chronic inflammation that is making you vulnerable to disease, as well as causing pain in your joints as you age. As a result, you will be healthier, live longer, and be able to move and exercise in the fat-burning, muscle-building ways you were genetically designed for.

PRIMAL EATING AND INFLAMMATION

We have seen how the human body, genetically speaking, is the same today as it was more than 2 million years ago, when we were Paleolithic hunter-gatherers. Then, our diet consisted of high-quality animal protein that was hormone, antibiotic, and pesticide free. The meat from animals our ancestors hunted was naturally organic and completely grass-fed, meaning the animals grazed on open ranges and ate wild grasses. This yielded a diet high in fat, a valued nutrient, because fat is the most dense form of energy.

You have seen how eating a high-carbohydrate meal increases blood sugar and stimulates the production of insulin, causing fat to be deposited in fat cells. But eating high-carbohydrate foods can also increase pro-inflammatory hormones, which inflame the body and lead to a large number of diseases.

The Primal Diet is naturally low in carbohydrates, so it reduces chronically elevated insulin levels in the body. Additionally, it is high in omega-3, the anti-inflammatory fatty acid, and low in omega-6, the pro-inflammatory fatty acid, so it improves your omega-6 to omega-3 ratio (more on omega-3s and -6s on pages 72 and 75). This kind of diet is highly effective for reducing chronic levels of inflammation. When you have less inflammation in your body, you feel more like moving and exercising.

It's important to keep in mind that we evolved on very few carbohydrates, because carbohydrate foods, mostly derived from fibrous vegetables and leafy greens, were scarce in Paleolithic times. A diet relying heavily on grains—bread, cereals, flour, and sweetened processed foods—is relatively new to our genome and therefore doesn't work congruently with our inherited physiology.

INFLAMMATION—WHAT IS IT AND HOW IT BECOMES CHRONIC

Inflammation is a normal part of your body's immune system. When you cut your finger, for example, white blood cells secrete a number of inflammation-promoting chemicals that rush to the injured area, where they fight germs and rid your body of damaged cells. Then, once the wound is healed, your immune system settles back down, no longer needing to respond with inflammatory substances.

But not always. Sometimes, the immune system stays active. Stress and dietary imbalances can confuse the body into thinking that it's under assault, even when there's no real threat. The result is a continued immune response, chronic inflammation, leading to systemic inflammation associated with many of the modern degenerative diseases.

Controlling inflammation not only reduces your risk for disease, it also decreases pain and stiffness in your joints, accelerates your recovery from injury and improves your overall mobility. Increased mobility equates with increased exercise, resulting in more success at weight loss. It also helps you to age gracefully, avoiding the bent postures and jerky movements that make you look older and less functional than you actually are.

Chronic inflammation has many causes. One cause is a diet consisting of foods high in "bad" fats—omega-6 essential fatty acids (EFAs). Let's look first at how bad or toxic fats can make inflammation skyrocket in your body, causing painful joints that contribute to your becoming sedentary, gaining weight, and experiencing other degenerative conditions.

Barry Sears, PhD, author of *The Zone*, wrote about how the modern-day diet is linked to chronic disease in his book *Toxic Fat: When Good Fats Turn Bad*. According to Sears, over the past few decades, three distinct dietary factors have come together to create what he calls the "perfect nutritional storm." These are (1) an increase in the consumption of cheap refined carbohydrates, which causes high insulin levels; (2) an increase in the use of cheap vegetable oils, which are high in pro-inflammatory omega-6 essential fatty acid; and (3) a decrease in the consumption of fish oils, which are high in anti-inflammatory omega-3 essential fatty acids.

Sears explains that when you consume an excess of cheap carbohydrates and cheap vegetable oils together, the increased levels of insulin from the carbohydrates cause the omega-6 essential fatty acids from the vegetable oils to produce arachidonic acid (AA), a powerful inflammatory hormone. This results in a constant low-level of inflammation that develops into chronic disease. Sears theorizes that AA, which he calls "toxic fat," is the underlying cause of chronic disease; it provides the linkage between obesity and chronic diseases, such as diabetes.

A healthy balance of omega-3 to omega-6 EFAs is important for keeping inflammation under control. Prior to agriculture, the omega-6/omega-3 EFA ratio ranged from 1 to 1 to 3 to 1. Modern-day omega-6/omega-3 EFA ratios average about 20 to 1. In evolutionary history, it was the adoption of agriculture that created a significant change in omega-6/omega-3 EFA ratios, because grains are high in omega-6 EFAs. Other dietary changes that occurred at this time included the introduction of cold-pressed oils, (such as corn, sunflower, and safflower, which are predominately omega-6) and the use of commercially raised animals that were fed grain instead of grass. All these dietary changes contributed to unnaturally high omega-6/omega-3 EFA ratios.

There is little doubt that the foods you eat directly influence the level of inflammation in your body, or as it's recently been coined, *inflamm-aging*, because as you age, you are more likely to have chronic inflammation—an association that could be causative. Foods affect hormones, and hormones are powerful substances in the body, sending messages that determine whether and when your immune response is turned on or off. What you eat is directly linked to how much inflammation is in your body.

GUIDELINES TO KEEP INFLAMMATION LOW

You can help control chronic levels of inflammation in your body by following these important guidelines:

Eat good fat, not bad fat. As I have said, hormones regulate inflammation, and your body manufactures hormones using essential fatty acids. They are considered essential, because the body cannot manufacture them on its own; they must be obtained from the food you eat. The omega-3 essential fatty acids (EFAs) are anti-inflammatory, and the omega-6 essential fatty acids are pro-inflammatory.

An anti-inflammatory diet includes lots of foods rich in omega-3, such as Alaskan salmon, herring, mackerel, wild game, grass-fed meats, omega-3-enriched eggs and dark leafy greens. To be avoided are foods that contribute pro-inflammatory omega-6 EFAs, found in grains and many of the vegetable oils, such as safflower, sunflower, corn, and soybean. Omega-6 fatty acids can also be found in most processed and fried foods, because those foods contain vegetable oils.

Wild animals that graze on grass are leaner than grain-fed farm animals, so their meat is leaner, although still high in fat. Grass-fed meat has a different fatty acid profile than grain-fed does. The majority of the meat we eat, if we don't shop at Whole Foods or other natural food stores, is grain-fed, so it's high in omega-6 EFAs and high in saturated fat. That's what happens when you feed animals grains instead of grass.

Grass-fed beef is a very different product from the beef normally sold in American grocery stores. The latter meat comes from cattle penned up in large feedlots where they are confined, fed grains, treated with hormones, and given antibiotics, all to promote fast weight gain and prevent diseases that are so prevalent in this unnatural environment.

Grass-fed meat is higher in anti-inflammatory omega-3 EFAs and lower in saturated fat than grain-fed meat is. It has a different fatty acid profile, but is still high in fat overall, and that's where ancestral humans got the majority of their fat, as well as the majority of their nutrients, because fat is so dense. Protein has 4 calories per gram, carbohydrate has 4 calories per gram, and fat has 9 calories per gram. Our ancestors got most of their nutrients from fat, so as a species, we are naturally fat eaters.

Good Fats/Bad Fats

(adapted from *The Protein Power Lifeplan* of the Drs. Eades)

GOOD FATS to include in your diet:

For cooking: Butter, ghee, olive oil, sesame seed oil, coconut oil, lard (natural and organic), and fat that occurs in natural meats and poultry

For baking: Almond oil, butter, ghee, and lard (natural and organic)

For salads: Avocado oil, almond oil, hazelnut oil, macadamia nut oil, olive oil, sesame seed oil, walnut oil, and flaxseed oil

BAD FATS to avoid in your diet:

Vegetable cooking oils (corn, soy, canola, safflower, sunflower), margarine, vegetable shortening, and partially hydrogenated oils of any kind

---

The Primal diet requires that you consume animal protein and fat from clean, grass-fed, organic sources free of industrial pesticides and hormones. Most toxins are fat soluble and will store easily in animal fat, transferring those toxins into your own body and making animal fat a "bad" fat, not good for consumption, unless you stick with "grass-fed, free-range" labeled products.

Eat a variety of plant food. Wild plants consumed by hunter-gatherers had high micronutrient concentrations. To replicate their diet, eat an abundance of plant foods that provide vitamins, minerals, fiber, and phytonutrients—all important to your health. The best sources are locally grown, organic, and in season such as the produce found at your local farmers' market.

It's no secret that vegetables and fruits are good for us. You may assume that it is because they contain minerals and vitamins, but plants are also rich in phytonutrients, certain organic compounds that help protect the plant from environmental damage, such as from ultraviolet light. Phytonutrients have a similar protective quality for us, too, in helping the body to repair damaged cells, build up the immune system, and act as powerful antioxidants. Many of the health benefits are believed to come from the different chemical compounds that give them their vibrant colors, which is why it important to include the five categories of plant colors in your diet: green, white, blue/purple, red, and yellow/orange.

Green plants (green beans, avocados, green peppers, and leafy greens) are rich in lutein, a carotenoid that is helpful for vision. *White* plants (onions, garlic, leeks, shallots, and chives) contain compounds that suppress tumor formation. *Blue/purple plants* (blueberries, broccoli, plums, and eggplant) contain powerful anti-oxidants which protect against cancer and reduce inflammation. *Red plants* (tomatoes, beets, chard, and strawberries) contain lycopene, which reduces harmful free radicals. *Yellow/orange* plants (carrots, golden bell peppers, oranges, and lemons) contain beta-carotene, which enhances the immune system.

Keep sugar low, including fruit. Although you want to get an abundance of plant food in your diet, eat fruits moderately on the Primal diet. Most people think of fruits as healthy and natural, and certainly the wild fruit that our Paleolithic ancestors ate was healthy, but their fruit was more tart and fibrous than the sweet, plump, and highly cultivated varieties available today. In addition, fruit in Paleolithic times was only seasonally available, which naturally limited amounts available in the diet.

The problem with fruit is that although fructose (fruit sugar), may not cause a rise in insulin (because the body metabolizes it differently than other sugar), it is extremely glycating. Andrew Weil discusses the "glycation theory of aging" in his book *Healthy Aging* and likens the process of glycation to carmelization, the process of sugar browning when heated. He suggests that a kind of carmelization happens in the body when there's enough sugar present in the blood, gumming up adjacent proteins and forming advanced glycation end products (AGEs). AGEs are deformed proteins that promote inflammation—and the acronym helps us remember the negative effect of modern diet on longevity and health.

Glycation from fructose happens more than from other forms of sugar, such as glucose or the ubiquitous table sugar. In addition, studies have shown that consuming large quantities of fructose (also found as high-fructose corn syrup in many processed foods) can ultimately impair your body's ability to handle glucose, leading to the negative condition of insulin resistance. Some of the sweeter fruits to avoid include bananas, grapes, dates, pineapple, watermelon, cantaloupe, kiwi, and raisins. Better fruit choices include apples, pears, strawberries, blackberries, raspberries, grapefruit, plums, lemons, and limes.

Avoid grains and legumes (beans). Almost all grains and legumes contain anti-nutrients, such as lectins and saponins. Lectins are sugar proteins that provide a protective barrier for the plant. When plants are attacked by parasites or mold, for example, lectins attach themselves to the invading cells to block the attack and, in the process, render the sugar molecules useless. This may be great for plants, but when you eat foods that contain lectins, they travel through your digestive tract and attach themselves to healthy sugar molecules needed for digestion. Those sugars are then viewed as defective and attacked by your immune system. This can lead to intestinal permeability and increased risk of inflammatory disease. Most legumes also contain saponins, which are known to disrupt cell membranes and lead to altered or damaged intestinal lining, causing "leaky gut syndrome."

Consume fresh, raw nuts and seeds in your diet, in small amounts. Nuts and seeds are a great snack food; they are tasty, easy to carry, and loaded with vitamins and minerals. The best choices are macadamia nuts, almonds, pecans, Brazil nuts, pistachios, walnuts, and hazelnuts, as well as pumpkin, sunflower, and sesame seeds.

One caveat: Nuts and seeds contain an antinutrient, phytic acid, which binds to minerals and prevents their absorption. Also, many contain a high proportion of omega-6 fatty acid, so you want to keep your consumption to a minimum.

Include dairy, in small amounts, if tolerated. While dairy is technically not a Paleolithic food, the Weston A. Price Foundation argues that raw dairy is perfectly nourishing, so it falls in the gray area.

Dairy is loaded with beneficial bacteria, protein, essential fatty acids, saturated fats, and some carbs. The best choices are full-fat, cultured milk products, such as yogurt and kefir, which introduce beneficial probiotics into the gut; raw butter, and cream, which are full of saturated fat; and hard cheeses made from unpasteurized milk. If you decide to consume dairy, make sure the animals are grass-fed and look for organic, hormone, and antibiotic free sources.

Use the glycemic index/glycemic load. One way to assess the sugary content of foods is to use the glycemic index (GI), a measurement of how fast a carbohydrate food raises your blood sugar after you eat it. Remember, when your blood sugar rises quickly, the brain signals your pancreas to secrete insulin to lower blood sugar, converting excess sugar to fat for storage. The greater the increase in blood sugar, the more insulin your pancreas releases to drive blood sugar down, and, consequently, the more fat gets stored.

A food with a low GI will cause a small rise in blood sugar, while a food with a high GI will trigger a larger spike in blood sugar. A GI of 70 or more is considered high; whereas a GI of 55 or less is low. Some foods with higher GIs are whole wheat bread at 75, cornflakes at 81, and baked potatoes at 85. Healthier choices include raw apples with a GI of 36, Greek yogurt with a GI of 12, and raw carrots with a GI of 35. Another point to consider is that meals containing protein and fat will cause a much lower spike in blood sugar than a heavily carbohydrate meal, because they slow down digestion, thereby lowering the meal's overall GI.

Another relatively new measurement, based on the GI, takes into account the amount of carbohydrate per serving, rather than solely the sugar in the food. This is called the glycemic load (GL). GL is calculated by dividing the GI by 100, and multiplying the result by the grams of carbohydrate per serving. As a reference, a GL of 20 or more is considered high; while a GL of 10 or less is low. Watermelon, for example, has a high GI but a relatively low GL. This is because in a typical serving of watermelon, there are only 6 grams of carbohydrate, bringing the GL measurement to about 4 on the scale.

The bottom line is choosing carbohydrates based on their GL is better than choosing them based only on their GI. Ultimately, you want to lower the starch and sugar content of your diet as much as possible. A good online reference for the GI and GL of foods is located at www.mendosa.com/gilists.htm.

THE DRUG OF CHOICE FOR EARLY HUMANS

Recognizing the problems created by a diet heavy in carbohydrate foods, I've often wondered why early humans ever wanted to become farmers. In hindsight, the transition from the hunter-gatherer lifestyle to agriculture has been celebrated as a major advance in civilization. But before civilization, hunter-gathering humans had no idea what was to come or where they were headed. Theirs was a good life. Scientists tell us that they worked about seventeen hours a week, leaving plenty of time for leisure, enjoyed near perfect health, and lived long, healthy lives when not killed by predators or natural disasters.

So why would anyone choose to become a farmer, when planting and field work required toiling from sun up to sundown? In addition, the changeover to the agricultural diet resulted in many nutritional deficiencies, because farmers no longer consumed the large variety of nutrient-rich plant foods they'd previously foraged; they relied on only one or two crops for nourishment. Agriculture also meant that people were now sedentary, and so more vulnerable to infectious disease and epidemics, because they lived in large groups in relatively small geographic areas. In general, as agriculture evolved as a lifestyle, the quality of life our early ancestors had at one time enjoyed declined considerably.

One of the more compelling theories to explain the changeover is presented in an article that appeared in the journal *Australian Biologist,* "The Origins of Agriculture: A Biological Perspective and a New Hypothesis." The authors suggest that humans invented agriculture so they could experience the euphoria produced by grains and dairy products. The idea is that grains and dairy products contain certain pharmacological substances called exorphins that affect humans the way opium does.

The authors report that "the ingestion of cereals and milk, in normal modern dietary amounts by normal humans, activates reward centers in the brain. Foods that were common in the diet before agriculture (fruits and so on) do not have this pharmacological property. The effects of exorphins are qualitatively the same as those produced by other opioid and/or dopaminergic drugs—that is, reward, motivation, reduction of anxiety, a sense of wellbeing, and perhaps even addiction. Though the effects of a typical meal are quantitatively less than those of doses of those drugs, most modern humans experience them several times a day, every day of their adult lives."[1]

Is it fair to say that as a species, we humans got "hooked" on agricultural and domesticated foods, tilling the fields to make sure we got our daily fix of exorphins? An intriguing idea, and as there are no cogent theories as to why early humans took to farming, I like this one as a way to understand why a behavior that seems irrational became the norm for our early human ancestors.

The good news is that you can kick this addiction to grains and products from domesticated animals and become much healthier.

DISPELLING THE MYTHS

The diet our ancestors ate kept their body inflammation and pain free, able to move with ease and perform fat-burning, muscle-strengthening kinds of activity patterns. However, the introduction of low-carbohydrate, high-fat, and high-protein diets (the Atkins diet, South Beach diet, and the Drs. Eades' Protein Power diet, to mention a few) to the general public have met with some loud objections. Most of the controversy surrounding the low-carb diet is based on three myths that I will dispel, relying on the latest scientific research about how diet impacts health.

Myth #1: Eating saturated fat from animal protein causes heart disease.
The first myth surrounding the low-carb diet approach is called the diet-heart hypothesis. This is the false idea that eating saturated fat from animal protein raises your cholesterol, specifically your LDL and total cholesterol, to clog your arteries and cause heart disease. It was the late Ancel Keys who convinced us that dietary fat causes heart disease. He became famous for developing the K ration for combat troops during World War II. Throughout the 1950s, Keys insisted that all fat, both vegetable and animal, raised cholesterol levels. This was how we came to believe that a low-fat diet is a healthy diet.

One of the most influential studies often cited as proof of the diet-heart hypothesis is known as the Framingham Heart Study, conducted under the direction of the National Heart, Lung and Blood Institute. Set up by Harvard University Medical School in 1948, this study involved 5,100 local residents divided into two groups: those who consumed little cholesterol and saturated fat in their diet and those who consumed large amounts of those substances. These groups were re-examined every five years to see which had the most heart disease.

After forty years, the director of this study, Dr. William Castelli, made the following admission: "In Framingham, Mass, the more saturated fat one ate, the more cholesterol one ate, the more calories one ate—the lower the person's serum cholesterol. . . . We found that the people who ate the most cholesterol, ate the most saturated fat, ate the most calories, weighed the least and were the most physically active."[2]

One of the researchers of the Framingham Heart Study, George V. Mann, commented, "On-going issues of pride, profit and prejudice caused outdated and never proven notions of the saturated fat/cholesterol hypothesis to persist, despite a lack of supportive evidence in the medical literature."

Mary Enig, consulting editor to the *Journal of the American College of Nutrition* and president of the Maryland Nutritionists Association, in addition to being a world-renowned lipids researcher, states, "The idea that saturated fats cause heart disease is completely wrong, but the statement has been published so many times over the last three or more decades that it is very difficult to convince people otherwise, unless they are willing to take the time to read and learn what produced the anti-saturated fat agenda."

The pharmaceutical and vegetable oil industries vilified saturated fat and were involved in promoting the research that supported the antisaturated fat agenda, as they had much to gain in the way of profits. What started out as a plausible theory has never been proven, despite the millions of dollars that were spent. As a result, people are confused and misinformed about the relation between diet and heart disease.

However, when you consider the high saturated fat content advised in the Primal diet, results are more supportive of the Framingham study results, rather than the recommendations of food and drug companies with an interest in selling cheap foods competitively and drugs that answer a need that is completely manufactured.

Understanding what is going on with HDL and LDL cholesterol and low-carb diets can also go far in dispelling the diet-heart hypothesis. A recent study compared the effects of a very low-carbohydrate, high-saturated-fat diet with a low-fat diet to evaluate long-term weight loss over a one-year period. The outcome of the study was that the low-carb group lost more weight and had greater decreases in triglycerides and increases in HDL cholesterol—the "good" kind—but there was also a minor increase in their LDL, or "bad" cholesterol.

According to what most doctors advise, an increase in LDL is dangerous, because LDL is known as the bad stuff that clogs arteries and causes heart disease. But that is up for question. Dr. Michael Eades points out on his blog that "numerous studies have shown that whenever subjects go on low-carb diets, they end up increasing the size of their LDL particles. Large, fluffy LDL particles are not only harmless, but may be protective. If they are protective, what's wrong with having a bit more of them?"[3]

Cholesterol is a soft, waxy substance found in every cell of the human body. It is especially abundant in cell membranes, where it helps maintain the integrity of these membranes; it also plays a role in cell signaling so that your cells can communicate with one another; and it helps the body produce hormones, bile acid, and vitamin D.

Because cholesterol does not dissolve in the blood, it is attached to a lipoprotein that transports it and then dissolves with it. Lipoproteins are classified according to their density. High-density lipoproteins (HDL) carry cholesterol away from the arteries and transport it to the liver to be excreted from the body in bile. Low-density lipoproteins (LDL) deposit cholesterol on the artery walls, which can lead to a narrowing of the arteries, called atherosclerosis, and increases the risk for heart disease.

Within the category of LDL, researchers have found that not all particles are created equal. When viewed under an electron microscope, some LDL particles appear large and fluffy, while others appear small and dense. Surprisingly, the big, fluffy LDL particles are harmless, whereas the small, dense particles do more damage. The reason is that the small, dense particles can fit between the cells that line the inner wall of the arteries. They are also more easily oxidized, which plays a role in forming cholesterol plaques, which can result in a heart attack. The bottom line is that LDL particle size predicts the risk for heart disease more accurately than does simply measuring total LDL cholesterol.

One more point is that small, dense LDL particles are strongly correlated with high triglycerides, or fat in the blood, and vice versa. Large, fluffy LDL particles correlate with low triglyceride levels. So if your triglycerides are low, which happens when you eat the low-carb ancestral diet, your LDL particles are probably large, fluffy, and harmless.

In my opinion . . . the lipid parameters of most value in determining risk for heart disease are triglyceride levels and HDL levels. In fact an important index of risk is the triglyceride to HDL ratio (TGL/HDL): the lower the better.

—DR. MICHAEL R. EADES

Myth #2: A diet of animal products causes loss of bone density. The osteoporosis threat is the second most common objection to the low-carb, high-protein diet. The question arises: Does eating too much meat cause leaching of calcium from bones?

Everything you eat when metabolized releases either an acid or an alkaline by-product into the blood. Animal protein releases an acid by-product, creating a mild, metabolic acidosis in your body. This excess acid is buffered by calcium leached from the bones, causing a loss of bone density. The answer is therefore yes—eating too much meat can cause bone loss, leading to osteoporosis, *unless* you eat enough calcium-rich foods to provide a buffer, effectively neutralizing the acidosis.

Understanding how calcium is handled in your body is the key to dispelling the myth that eating meat will cause bone loss. Nutritionists tell us that there is a balance between how much calcium you take in and how much you excrete, known as the calcium balance. It's quite possible to take in a lot of calcium and still be low in calcium, if your excretion is high. It's also possible to take in very little calcium and be in calcium balance, if you excrete very little calcium.

The main factor that determines how much calcium is excreted is the acid–alkaline balance in your blood. So the best way to neutralize acid-forming foods (animal products) and retain more calcium is to eat more alkaline foods. Most plant foods—dark leafy greens, colorful vegetables, and low-glycemic fruits—create a mild alkalosis in the blood, and so buffer acid-forming foods.

Grains, dairy products, legumes, meat, fish, and eggs all produce acid. Surprisingly, hard cheeses are the most acidic of all. You would think that cheese would help build strong bones, because it is rich in calcium, but unless you consume enough plant foods, the excess acid could cause bone loss.

On a short-term basis, our body can handle an acid buildup and the amount of calcium lost from the bones would not be of any consequence. What we are talking about is if this mild acidosis goes on for decades. That would eventually lead to osteoporosis. But protecting your bones is easy if you follow the low-carb Primal diet, which is rich in alkalizing (acid-buffering) plant foods. Other factors for maintaining bone density include taking a calcium supplement, getting plenty of sunshine, and taking additional vitamin D to help with the absorption of calcium. This will ensure strong, healthy bones!

Myth #3: Too much protein can damage your kidneys. A final myth is that of the threat of kidney disease. Although studies have shown that in individuals with

Exercise and Bone Density

Two types of exercises impact bone health: resistance exercises and weight-bearing exercises. RESISTANCE EXERCISE refers to the use of free weights or body weight exercises to strengthen the muscles and the bones to which they attach. WEIGHT-BEARING refers to exercises in which your bones and muscles work against gravity. Sprinting, walking, and stair climbing are all examples of weight-bearing exercises. Aerobic exercises, such as swimming and bicycling, are not considered weight bearing.

Numerous research studies have shown that the effect of resistance exercise is relatively site specific to the muscles worked and the bones to which the muscles attach. Also, although aerobic weight-bearing activity is important in maintaining overall health and healthy bone, resistance training has a more potent impact on bone density. In particular, high-intensity resistance training has the best effect—considering our genetic inheritance and how using our fast-twitch muscle fibers give us an evolutionary advantage.

preexisting unhealthy kidneys, excessive protein may indeed cause undue strain on this organ, there's not one scientific study, using healthy adults with normal kidney function, showing excessive protein causes kidney damage.

In fact, quite the contrary. In one study, researchers examined the renal (kidney) function of bodybuilders and other well-trained athletes with a high- and medium-protein diet. The athletes underwent a seven-day nutrition record analysis, as well as blood samples and urine collection, to see whether these diets affected kidney function. The study found that both groups of athletes had renal clearances that were within the normal range, concluding that "there were no correlations between protein intake and creatinine clearance, albumin excretion rate, and calcium excretion rate." In other words, a high-protein diet does not impair kidney function in well-trained athletes, at least in the short term.

In another study, researchers investigated the effect of protein intake on renal function in 1,624 women between the ages of forty-two and sixty-eight enrolled in the Nurses' Health Study over an eleven-year period. The researchers concluded that "high protein intake was not associated with renal function decline in women with normal renal function."[4]

From a purely anecdotal point of view, athletes and bodybuilders have been known to consume high-protein diets for long periods of time. If a high-protein diet caused kidney damage, you would expect to see kidney problems showing up in this group. But that has not happened, suggesting that these diets are not harmful to the kidneys.

One caveat: When choosing protein sources, always choose organic, grass-fed meat, free-range poultry, and wild fish whenever possible. Although healthy kidneys should have no trouble processing high-quality meats, many of the animal protein sources available in our modern world are highly toxic and could burden anyone's kidneys. Plus, most supermarket/butcher-bought meat is far removed from the wild animals our ancestors ate, and therefore not in congruence with our genetic blueprint.

EAT PRIMAL: FIVE SIMPLE TIPS

In Chapter 9, I will help you design a meal plan for an easy and convenient adaptation to the Primal diet. Here are five easy-to-remember main points, to get you started. Keeping these tips in mind will naturally move you in the right direction toward more Primal eating habits and align your diet with the natural expression of your DNA.

1. **Focus your meals on high-quality animal protein,** such as fresh beef, fish, and poultry. Whenever possible, consume local, grass-fed, free-range, organic, antibiotic, pesticide and hormone-free meat, which has a healthier fat profile.

2. **Eat an abundance of plant foods,** such as brightly colored vegetables, berries, and low-glycemic fruit, which are rich in vitamins, minerals, antioxidants, and phytonutrients. Many of the health benefits are believed to come from the chemical compounds that give them their vibrant colors.

3. **Include fresh, raw nuts and seeds in your diet,** such as walnuts, macadamia nuts, almonds, pecans, hazelnuts, Brazil nuts, and pistachios, as well as pumpkin, sesame, and sunflower seeds.

4. **Avoid all processed, fried, and fast foods,** including most snack foods, baked goods, frozen meals, and sweets. They are high in refined carbohydrates, bad fats, and sweeteners, and low in vitamins, minerals, and nutrients.

5. **Avoid vegetable oils,** such as corn, soy, canola, safflower, and sunflower oils, as well as mayonnaise, margarine, and shortening, and increase consumption of all foods high in omega-3 fatty acids, especially from fish.

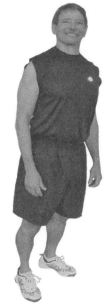

Ron's Transformation
Getting Pain-Free and Moving Once Again

RON, a fifty-eight-year-old social investor/entrepreneur, came to me when his wife, who I'd been training, recommended he get help with issues that were preventing him from working as hard as he wanted to stay fit. I'll let him describe the painful condition he'd been dealing with, and how he benefited from all five steps of my program to become fit and pain free after years of limitation.

I've been working out and playing sports most of my life. I have a small boat and race it extensively at the national and world levels, so in order to maintain my strength and agility, I've been doing yoga, weight lifting, and as much as possible getting cardio in by running and biking.

But over the last ten to fifteen years, I've had to give up running, because after every run I'd be in pain for a number of days. My knees were in bad shape, due to old basketball and lacrosse injuries. Over the years, the injuries led to me making compensatory adjustments to minimize the movements of my knees, while at the same time, developing movement patterns that seemed to make my knees more injury-prone. I took up bike riding, but it soon got to the point where even that was causing continued inflammation of my knees.

About a year ago, one knee was particularly bad, and I was in constant pain from what had deteriorated to a bone-on-bone condition with a lot of inflammation. Even though I'd had several surgeries on that knee, it was continuing to get worse. I was diagnosed as being in a stage 4 condition, and the next step I was told would be the onset of arthritis and a big reduction in mobility. That was the last straw, and I decided to see what Mikki's program could offer.

My goal in starting to train was to get back to where I was pain free—to have increased mobility and be able to do things I hadn't been able to do, like ride a bike. It was beyond my dreams to think I might ever run again! But what I learned from Mikki was how to address the underlying issue that was causing my knees to get worse—in spite of all I'd done to fix and protect them—which was me using my knees in the wrong way.

To begin with, Mikki got me using the foam roller to keep my muscles loose so they could function better. Working out on tight muscles was not helping me, but instead was making my muscles even tighter and not building the strength and flexibility I wanted. So using the foam roller before working out made my progress faster.

In my diet, I'd been gradually moving away from eating high carbs, but today I eat mostly protein, vegetables, and fruits, following the Paleo diet as prescribed by Mikki.

Supplementing my diet also helped. With the reduced inflammation and the change in how I worked out, my knees started to feel much better.

But the biggest change was in the way I moved and used my knees. I learned some basic, Primal movement patterns that corrected the compensations I'd developed over the years from having pain and lack of mobility in my knees. We worked on getting my knees to do what knees were supposed to do and make other parts of my body, particularly my hips, do what they were supposed to do—back to functioning in ways that made things better, not worse. For example, learning to hinge, using my hips, actually minimized the work my knees had to do, and adopting that new pattern greatly relieved the stress on my knees and the resulting pain.

We also worked on exercises to strengthen muscles that would improve the use of my hips. As a result, I was able to establish more functional ways of walking, of standing, of using my legs, than I'd been able to do for so many years.

Now I'm running again, but this time it's up and down stadium steps, and now I'm adding intensity by doing intervals on the stairs. And I'm on a bike again, without any inflammation or pain afterward!

What makes the program so successful for me was the multipronged approach: correcting movement patterns, bringing the inflammation down with supplements and diet, and loosening and strengthening the quads and glutes—all of which helped me to use my knees in the way that no longer creates pain today.

My original goals—to build strength, learn new movement habits, and get rid of the pain—have all been met. Focusing on keeping the supplements and diet going, gradually getting stronger and trying new things—all of that has made the difference in me living and exercising with a renewed sense of my capabilities—and remaining pain free.

NEXT . . .

In the next step, you will learn how early humans had no need to take vitamins or minerals in supplement form, but you, as a modern human, do. When you supplement your diet with key nutrients, you match the nutrient density they enjoyed naturally in their Primal diets, so it's important to know exactly how to do that.

STEP 1

Chapter 5

Step Two—Supplement with the Super Six

The image of cavemen and -women, sitting around the fire eating a mammoth thigh, stopping to take their vitamins might be the stuff of a funny cartoon, the scene being so incongruous for obvious reasons. But the reality is that early humans had no need to supplement their diet—it was that good!

Our ancestors ate foods high in protein and fat, and low in carbohydrates, the exact opposite of most modern humans' diets today. But dietary content is not the only thing that was different back then. Nutrient density, meaning the actual vitamins, minerals, and other essential nutrients contained in their food—was different, too. Paleo-anthropologists have shown us that the foods our ancestors ate had greater nutrient density, even when comparing the same food to the food we are eating today.

For example, the vitamin and mineral content of our steak, apple, or carrot can't stand up to similar foods that our ancestors ate, as the following chart of contemporary hunter-gatherer nutrient intake shows.

Comparative Hunter-Gatherer Nutrient Intake[1]

NUTRIENT	PALEOLITHIC INTAKE	RDA	U.S. INTAKE
Vitamin C	604 mg	60 mg	77–109 mg
Vitamin E	33 mg	8–10 mg	7–10 mg
Calcium	1,956 mg	800–1,200 mg	750 mg
Magnesium	700 mg	350 mg	250 mg
Potassium	10,500 mg	3,500 mg	2,500 mg
Zinc	43 mg	12–15 mg	5–14 mg
Fiber	50–104 g	25–35 g	10 g

Why was our ancestors' food so much more nutritionally dense than ours is today? For one, the soil in which their food grew was not as depleted as our soil is today, due to modern farming methods that strip vital minerals through over-planting. Even if you shop at the local farmers' market and buy organic food, you are not getting the same quality of nutrients as our ancestors got from their mineral-rich soils. Also, they didn't have to deal with the huge amount of environmental toxins, as well as the chronic stress that challenges modern bodies. For these reasons, they managed to function optimally and stay clear of the diseases of civilization so endemic today, such as heart disease, diabetes, and cancer.

To match the nutrient density of the foods our ancestors ate, we modern humans need to supplement our diet with the right vitamins, minerals, and other substances that I recommend in this chapter. My list of Super Six Supplements will ensure that you are getting the same amount and quality of nourishment from your food that your DNA evolved on for millions of years, fulfilling your genetic blueprint that determines how you stay lean, fit, and healthy at any age.

SUPPLEMENTS AND FAT-LOSS BENEFITS

When you take supplements to match the density of the ancestral diet, you not only become healthier, you eliminate constantly feeling hungry and tired. This translates directly to you eating less and having more energy to exercise, thereby gaining more muscle and losing more fat. In addition, when your diet is supplemented correctly for your DNA, you won't be loaded with painful inflammation, slowing you down and discouraging you from doing the kinds of activity that burns fat. You will begin to feel healthier and be more energetic, less likely to lapse into sedentary habits and more likely to perform natural activity.

Once again, modern scientific research confirms the wisdom of living congruent to our genetic inheritance. A new study published in the *International Journal of Obesity*, done by Chinese researchers, showed that a low-dose multivitamin-mineral caused obese volunteers to lose 7 lbs (3.2 kg) of fat in six months. In this study, ninety-six obese women aged eighteen through fifty-five were given either a multivitamin-mineral supplement, calcium, or a placebo during a twenty-six-week period. The researchers found that those who were given the multivitamin-mineral supplement lost more body weight and had a lower body mass index at the end of the study than did the others, without changing their regular diet.

Why would this be so? The authors suggested that the reason the women lost the weight was that obese people, in general, tend to have lower blood concentrations or lower bioavailability of a number of nutrients, including vitamins A, D, K, and several B vitamins; zinc; and iron, and that this could affect appetite. They also suggested that there was the possibility of increased calorie and fat burning from some of the nutrients.[2]

In regard to supplements helping fat loss, it's important to keep in mind that there is no magic bullet. As much as we all want to take that one little pill to get rid of overeating, sedentism, and weight gain forever, no such supplement exists. You don't gain weight overnight, and you can't lose it overnight, either, although improving the nutrient density of your food may help. Supplements are not a magic bullet to fix a problem, but work in relationship to the other aspects of the Primal Body Program, which are exercise and diet.

Before I introduce you to the Super Six, I want to issue two important warnings about taking supplements.

1. ***Supplements cannot make up for a poor diet or an insufficient exercise program.*** It's dangerous to rely on supplements as substitutes or replacements for any part of your fitness program. The majority of the results you will get from following the Primal Body Program will come from sticking close to the ancestral diet, and exercising in a way that mimics ancestral movement patterns, including metabolic training. Think of supplements as *supplemental*, something that you take in addition to a healthy diet and exercise program.

2. ***All supplements are* not *created equal.*** Because the supplement industry is not regulated, sometimes dosages vary and ingredients may be contaminated. So look for reputable companies. A number of manufacturers offer unbiased lab testing as proof of the quality of their product; they send random batches of their supplements to unbiased labs for testing and then publish the results of those findings. This is the best proof of quality.

Another way to ensure quality is to check vitamin bottles for the United States Pharmacopoeia (USP), NSF International (NSF), or ConsumerLab.com (CL) seals. The USP and NSF are nonprofit groups that verify whether companies offer contamination-free products and use good manufacturing practices. Not every brand has the seals; some don't want to submit to the testing. But you can be sure those that do are reliable.

INTRODUCING THE SUPER SIX

My choice of supplements is based on what our modern body needs to best replicate the nutritionally dense diet our ancestral humans ate. Following is a list of the nutritional supplements I recommend, in order of importance. Adding these supplements on a daily basis is a vital component of the Primal Body Program, helping you to get lean, fit, and healthy.

1. Omega-3 essential fatty acid
2. Vitamin D$_3$
3. Antioxidants (vitamins C, E, and coenzyme Q10)
4. Magnesium
5. Multinutritional formula
6. Glucosamine

Super Supplement #1: Omega-3/Essential Fatty Acids

If you had to limit your supplement intake to just one supplement, the one I'd recommend over all the others is omega-3 essential fatty acid. You may recall from Chapter 4 that omega-3 is an essential fatty acid (EFA), meaning it is a kind of fat your body doesn't make and therefore must be gotten from the food you eat.

In replicating the early human diet, the inclusion of omega-3 fatty acid is what separates the Primal Body diet from other high-protein and high-fat, low-carbohydrate plans, such as the Atkins diet. This is because in my diet, the emphasis is on "good fats," and getting the right kind of fat, not just any kind of fat, as is recommended in other diets.

Unfortunately, omega-3 fatty acid is the single most deficient nutrient in our modern diet, and we pay a hefty price in having adapted to its absence in our evolution. The following disorders and symptoms are correlated to the deficiency of omega-3 essential fats in our foods today: ADD/HD, dyslexia, depression, weight gain, heart disease, allergies, arthritis, violence, memory problems, cancer, eczema, inflammatory diseases, diabetes, dry skin, dandruff, postpartum depression, alcoholism, Crohn's disease, irritable bowel syndrome, cirrhosis of the liver, PMS, hypoglycemia, carbohydrate/sweet cravings, noncancerous breast disease, ulcerative colitis, scleroderma, Sjögren's syndrome, hypertension, bipolar disorder, irritability, soft or brittle nails, lowered immunity/frequent infections, frequent urination, fatigue, dry unmanageable hair, hyperactivity, excessive thirst, dry eyes, poor wound healing, learning problems, alligator skin, patches of pale skin on cheeks, and cracked skin on heels or fingertips.[3]

What is the cause of this rampant omega-3 deficiency? With the adoption of agriculture, ancestral humans began to eat more grains, which are high in omega-6 fatty acids but not omega-3s. They also tended to eat less grass-fed meat, which is an important source of omega-3s. Another dietary change that occurred at that time was the use of commercially raised animals that were fed grain instead of grass. All of these changes caused an increase in omega-6 consumption and a decrease in dietary consumption of omega-3.

Many years later, after the advent of the "diet-heart hypothesis," which linked consumption of dietary fat to heart disease and other health problems, fats were so heavily demonized that many people began thinking that the best solution to the fat problem was to completely avoid fat. And they were right, to a point. There are some types of fat you do want to avoid, such as trans fats, a product of the food industry's tampering with natural fats to enhance shelf life of foods containing fats. But omega-3s are so important for your health that they have been named essential fatty acids, because your body needs them to perform important functions and cannot manufacture them on its own. Foods that are rich in omega-3 fatty acids include seafood from cold waters, such as salmon, herring, black cod, mackerel, and sardines. Other sources include wild game, including grass-fed beef, lamb, venison, and buffalo; omega-3 enriched eggs; walnuts; and dark leafy greens. (Chia seeds and flaxseeds are not great sources of omega-3 because they are not easily converted from ALA to EPA and DHA in the body.)

Supplemental sources and dosages: Fish oil is the best supplemental source of omega-3, and can be taken in either capsule form or liquid in a bottle. But how much do you need?

The truth is that both omega-3 and omega-6 essential fatty acids perform important functions in the body. To create health rather than disease, a balanced intake of both omega-3 and omega-6 fatty acids is required, which is what our ancestors had in their diet before the agricultural revolution and processed foods came along. The optimal ratio of omega-6 to omega-3 is believed to be within the range of 3 to 1 and 1 to 1. The current average from the modern diet is not even close to that optimal range; it is approximately 20 to 1!

Although scientists have not yet come up with a universal recommendation for the exact dosage of omega-3 needed on a daily basis, some guidelines were established in 1999 at the Workshop on the Essentiality of and Recommended Dietary Intakes for Omega-6 and Omega-3 Fatty Acids, held in Bethesda, Maryland, and reported in the *Journal of the American College of Nutrition*. The workshop participants agreed on the following guidelines, based on a 2,000-calorie/per day diet: For omega-6 (linoleic acid), intake was set at 4.44 grams per day with an upper limit of 6.67 grams per day, and for omega-3 (alpha-linolenic acid) intake was set at 2.22 grams per day with no upper limit.[4]

This recommendation sounds simple enough—2 to 1, omega-6 to omega-3. But when you consider that one tablespoon of safflower oil (as in one serving of commercial salad dressing) supplies 10 grams of omega-6, already exceeding the upper limit of 6.67 grams, you can see just how easy it is to lose the delicate balance called for. In addition to your salad dressing, all the processed and fast foods you eat are loaded with vegetable oils, even the so-called healthy ones, such as whole-grain cakes, cookies, crackers, and breads. These foods are therefore sources of omega-6, tipping the balance in a way that most consumers are completely unaware of.

In a recent nutritional study, researchers showed how mimicking the omega-6 to omega-3 ratio of ancestral humans leads to changes in gene expression that can bring about less allergic inflammation and autoimmune disorders. Researchers at the Wake Forest University School of Medicine took twenty-seven healthy people and fed them a special diet that was designed to reproduce the omega-6 to omega-3 fatty acid ratio of our caveman ancestors for five weeks. They then looked at the gene levels of immune messenger molecules that impact autoimmunity and allergy and found that many key signaling genes that promote inflammation were markedly reduced, when compared to a normal diet. This included a signaling gene for a protein called PI3K, a critical early step in autoimmune and allergic inflammation responses.[5]

More proof that the ancestral diet lowers inflammation! But what's new in this study is that it demonstrates that gene expression is the mechanism by which the omega fatty acids reduce inflammation.

Taking into account the high amounts of omega-6 fatty acids we are all getting, it is a good idea to increase the level of omega-3 supplementation above the bottom-line 2.22 grams recommended per day. Many nutritionists recommend dosages in the range of 6 to 8 grams per day.

And remember that we are striving for balance, so in addition to supplementing your diet with omega-3, you would want to eliminate grains, legumes, grain-fed meats, all vegetable oils (except olive and coconut oil), all commercially processed foods and baked goods, all commercial salad dressings, and all fast foods, to bring down your intake of omega-6 fatty acids. Of course, the easiest way to achieve this optimum ratio of omega-6 to omega-3 would be to follow the ancestral diet. (One word of caution, however: If you are taking medications, such as blood thinners, consult with your doctor before using fish oil, because this supplement can thin your blood.)

Super Supplement #2: Vitamin D

This quote from leading nutritional expert Dr. Michael Holick, in his book *The Vitamin D Solution*, says it all: "If I had to give you a single secret ingredient that could apply to the prevention—and treatment, in many cases—of heart disease, common cancers, stroke, infectious diseases from influenza to tuberculosis, type 1 and 2 diabetes, dementia, depression, insomnia, muscle weakness, joint pain, fibromyalgia, osteoarthritis, rheumatoid arthritis, osteoporosis, psoriasis, multiple sclerosis, and hypertension, it would be this: vitamin D."

Vitamin D is often thought of as the "sunshine vitamin," because the body manufactures it after exposure to sunshine. Most people believe that ten minutes of daily exposure will supply all the vitamin D the body needs. While it is true that the body can manufacture vitamin D from cholesterol in the skin when exposed to ultraviolet B (UV-B) sunlight, it is more difficult than you might think to obtain adequate vitamin D with such brief exposure.

The reason is that the amount of UV-B available has to do with the angle of the sun's rays; latitude and altitude affect the intensity of UV light. Unless you live in the tropics, the only way you can form adequate vitamin D is by sunning between ten AM and two PM during the summer months if you live in the northern latitudes (or during the winter months if you live in the southern latitudes) for 20 to 120 minutes, depending on your skin type and color. One more factor is that 85 percent of your body surface needs to be exposed, just as it was for ancestral humans who most likely dressed in animal skins and loincloths when out in the midday sun.

In most parts of the United States, there is insufficient sunlight to produce optimal levels of vitamin D during six months of the year or more. No doubt the safest way to obtain vitamin D is from natural sunlight, but for most people it would not be possible to get adequate vitamin D this way. Surprisingly, a viable alternative is tanning beds using UV-B bulbs.

Vitamin D can also be obtained though diet, mainly from fish and animal fats. Ancestral humans consumed an abundance of vitamin D foods, including intestines, organ meats, and the skin of animals they caught, as well as fatty fish and insects. But in our modern diet, we tend to avoid vitamin D–rich foods, such as kippers, sardines, mackerel, herring, and the yolk when eating eggs. We also remove the skin, organs, and fats from our meat, and so miss most of the vitamin D available in foods.

Supplemental sources and dosages: The obvious solution is to supplement, but how much should you take to supply your body with what it needs?

Nora Gedgaudas, in *Primal Body, Primal Mind,* discusses the idea that nutrients do not operate in a vacuum, but that there is a "complex system of interrelationships" in the body that should be considered. For example, she mentions that for every receptor on cells in the body for vitamin D, there are two receptors for vitamin A. To achieve health, a balance of these two nutrients would be necessary, because deficiencies of vitamin A can make vitamin D toxic at lower levels. And too much vitamin A can result in a vitamin D deficiency. One way to deal with this would be to take cod liver oil, which tends to be high in vitamin A but low in vitamin D, and supplement with vitamin D.

According to early evolutionary theorist Weston Price, dietary intake of vitamin D by ancestral humans was approximately 4,000 IU per day. This, of course, was in addition to the enormous amounts of vitamin D synthesized in the body from daily exposure to sunshine.[6]

There are two different types of vitamin D—D_2 and D_3. Vitamin D_2 is a synthetic plant form not easily absorbed by the body. This is the type that vegans prefer, because it contains no animal products. However, vitamin D_2 is highly supported by the drug industry, which owns the patent and manufactures most quantities commercially available, so these companies have an enormous financial stake in D_2 sales and production. It can be found in foods, in milk supplementation, and in prescription vitamin D drugs.

Vitamin D_3 is the animal-based natural form manufactured from the wool of sheep (the animals are not harmed by this process). This form is produced in the human body with sunlight, so it is the preferred way to supplement with vitamin D.

The Vitamin D Council, a nonprofit, educational corporation in the state of California, suggests that there are three ways for adults to ensure adequate levels of vitamin D:

1. Regularly receive midday sun exposure in the late spring, summer, and early fall, exposing as much of the skin as possible (being careful to never burn).
2. Regularly use a sun bed (avoiding sunburn) during the colder months.
3. Take 5,000 IU per day for 2 to 3 months, then obtain a 25-hydroxy vitamin D test. Adjust your dosage so that blood levels are between 50 and 80 ng/mL (or 125 and 200 nmol/L) year-round.[7]

You can order the 25-hydroxy vitamin D test online at www.directlabs.com without a doctor's visit.

The question of sunscreen: One more point is to avoid sunscreen, as most SPF sunscreens are manufactured with an omega-6 base, contain many carcinogenic chemicals, and block all of the UV-B light needed to synthesize vitamin D. For example, some products contain PABA, a substance that can be chemically altered by the sun's rays to cause cancer. Recognizing this problem, many manufacturers have used other blocking agents and removed the PABA. But how do we know that these other blockers don't also change into dangerous compounds when exposed to the sun's rays?

The solution is to use your own natural sun protection, which is the gradual buildup of pigment within the skin. With regular sun exposure in small doses, your body can build up pigment to protect from the sun's potentially cancerous effects. You want to get an abundance of sunshine, so cover up only with a hat and clothing or get out of the sun at the first sign of reddening until you build up a good tan.

For those who are afraid of the sun, you might want to consider that according to the Drs. Eades, vitamin D can slow down the development and spread of melanoma, as well as the development of breast cancer, colon cancer, and cancer of the prostrate. Understanding the role vitamin D plays in your protection from these forms of cancer, you don't want to avoid the sun, but be smart about your degree of exposure.

Super Supplement #3: Antioxidants

Ancient humans evolved on a diet that was based on wild plants, particularly green leafy vegetables and meat from wild animals. These vegetables provided antioxidant vitamins, minerals, and many phytochemicals with a variety of antioxidant properties. Their diet had an enormous variety of plant foods, each containing a unique blend of protective compounds to counter free radical damage and other oxidative stress.

But to understand the value of antioxidants, you want first to understand the effects of free radicals in the human body. A free radical is an atom with an unpaired electron. The nucleus of an atom is surrounded by a ring of paired electrons. Sometimes an atom loses an electron (referred to as oxidation), leaving the atom with an unpaired electron. The atom is then a free radical and is said to be highly reactive, setting off a chain reaction of damaging events in the search for an electron to fill its outer ring. Free radicals damage DNA, proteins, cell membranes, and other structures.

The presence of too many free radicals creates a condition called oxidative stress. Andrew Weil, in *Healthy Aging*, says that "oxidative stress is simply the total burden placed on organisms by the constant production of free radicals in the normal course of metabolism. . . ."

Free radicals are produced in the body in a number of ways, but the most common production occurs in the mitochondria (cellular oxygen furnaces) through the electron transport chain. This is significant, because this energy system is used to produce ATP (the energy currency of the cell) during aerobic metabolism. So when you spend endless hours doing aerobic exercise, you are actually increasing free radical production, oxidative stress, and the likelihood of aging more quickly over time.

To reduce oxidative stress, cut back on aerobic exercise and do more anaerobic exercise, such as interval training, as presented in Step 5 of the Primal Body Program. Also, include in your diet an abundance of plant foods, which are loaded with antioxidants and other beneficial properties. Our bodies have enzymes (antioxidants) that intercept free radicals, convert them to less harmful substances (water and oxygen), and remove them from the body. These antioxidants are derived from foods that are rich in vitamins and E and C.

According to the Drs. Eades, most of the powerful cancer-fighting nutrients in plants are not absorbed well without eating some fat with them. These include the carotenoids, found in colorful plants, and lycopene, found in tomatoes. So, when you make a salad, use extra-virgin olive oil (EVOO) in the dressing; or if you steam vegetables, drizzle some EVOO on them.

In addition to eating an abundance of fresh fruits and vegetables, the best antioxidation strategy is to supplement your diet with vitamins E and C, and coenzyme Q10.

VITAMIN E

Vitamin E is a powerful fat-soluble antioxidant. It can protect your skin from ultra-violet light, prevent cell damage from free radicals, allow your cells to communicate effectively, and help protect against prostate cancer and Alzheimer's disease. It also aids in the protection and metabolism of essential fatty acids, so it is a good idea to take it with fish oil. Good sources include mustard greens, chard, sunflower seeds, turnip greens, almonds, and spinach.

Supplemental sources and dosages: Vitamin E is not an isolated nutrient but a family of fat-soluble vitamins that includes alpha-, beta-, gamma-, and delta-tocopherols and tocotrienols. Look for a source that contains mixed tocopherols and tocotrienols. Supplement with 400 to 800 IUs daily.

VITAMIN C

Vitamin C, a water-soluble vitamin, is a highly effective antioxidant. Besides strengthening the immune system to help you fight colds, it can protect proteins, lipids, carbohydrates, and DNA from free radical damage. It also regenerates other antioxidants such as vitamin E. It is needed in the synthesis of carnitine, which is essential for the transport of fat into the mitochondria, so that it can be converted to energy (think fat loss). And it helps the body produce collagen, the connective tissue that holds everything together throughout the body. The list of benefits goes on and on.

Dietary sources include red bell peppers, oranges, apples, beets, grapefruit, lemons, pears, plums, strawberries, broccoli, Brussels sprouts, cantaloupe, cauli-flower, garlic, grapes, Swiss chard, collard greens, asparagus, raspberries, tomatoes, green beans, summer squash, carrots, blueberries, spinach, celery, apricots, onions, avocados, cucumbers, kale, and more. . . .

Supplemental source and dosage: In addition to eating an abundance of dietary sources of vitamin C, supplement with 500 to 1,000 mgs daily. Vitamin C can be taken as a powder or pill, in a buffered form, time-released, and a variety of combination formulas.

COENZYME Q10

CoQ10 is a coenzyme, meaning that it helps enzymes, acting as a catalyst for biological chemical reactions. It is involved in basic energy production for every cell in the body. This energy production takes place in the mitochondria through a series of chemical reactions along the electron transport chain where ATP (the energy currency of the cell) is produced. CoQ10 is the messenger between the enzymes of this chain. Without coQ10, there is no production of energy for the cell, and without energy there is no life!

Given the importance of this supplement, you would think that coQ10 would be more widely used in the United States. But it's the same old story, preventing its more widespread use. Because it is a natural substance, it cannot be patented, so the drug manufacturers are not able to make any money from producing it. Worse yet, it might compete with patented drugs with similar functions. In Japan, however, coenzyme Q10 is one of the most popular supplements on the market.

Coenzyme Q10 is also a potent, fat-soluble antioxidant. It is helpful with cardiovascular conditions, cancer, immune disorders, and periodontal disease. It can also boost energy and speed recovery from exercise. Dietary sources include organ meats such as heart, liver, and kidney, as well as sardines and mackerel.

Supplemental source and dosage: Supplement with 100 mg of coQ10 daily. For individuals over age forty, or for those who are affected by chronic disease, ubiquinol is more beneficial, because the body's ability to produce coQ10 and convert it into ubiquinol might be diminished. The dosage is the same for both.

Super Supplement #4: Magnesium

Magnesium is one of the most important minerals in the body, used in over 350 enzyme processes. Every cell in your body has magnesium in it, yet it is one of the most overlooked and depleted minerals in the modern diet.

From a Paleolithic point of view, studies show that early humans consumed 700 to 1,500 mg of magnesium per day, and an equal amount of calcium. Modern-day humans consume about the same amount of calcium but average 150 to 300 mgs of magnesium per day.

This is significant because the two minerals, calcium and magnesium, work together. Calcium remains outside the cell until it is needed to generate an electrical impulse, while magnesium remains inside the cell. An excess of calcium in the body can upset this balance, causing low levels of magnesium inside the cell and high levels of calcium, leading to hardening of tissues and resulting muscle contractions (spasms). High levels of calcium inside the smooth muscles of the coronary arteries, for example, can cause these smooth muscles to spasm, elevating blood pressure. Interestingly, the medication for high blood pressure is a calcium blocker, although magnesium could have the same effect without the added expense. Additionally, it's safer and more natural.

Some of the illnesses associated with magnesium deficiency include asthma, constipation, muscle cramps, PMS, fibromyalgia, depression, hypoglycemia, insulin resistance, kidney stones, chronic fatigue syndrome, anxiety, depression, migraine headaches, hypertension (high blood pressure), and heart disease, among others.

If magnesium is so important, why haven't you heard more about it? Once again, as a natural substance it can't be patented, and therefore there's no incentive for pharmaceutical companies to do lengthy and expensive studies to prove its effectiveness. Unfortunately, money and profit drive research. Without large, long-term, double-blind, placebo-controlled studies showing the effectiveness of magnesium in such things as lowering blood pressure, improving insulin resistance, or controlling asthma, very few doctors are recommending magnesium, and no drug companies are paying for expensive ads to let consumers know about it.

Compared to being aware of the importance of calcium, which has the megamillion-dollar dairy industry touting its benefits, the average consumer knows very little about magnesium. You'd have to have lived in a cave to not have heard that calcium builds strong bones!

The depletion of magnesium in our soils is one reason why our diet is so deficient in magnesium. When plants grow, they get their minerals from the soil. But when crops are grown year after year without giving the soil a chance to be replenished, the soil becomes depleted. Another factor is that fertilizers replenish the potassium and phosphorous but not the magnesium, so there's less magnesium in the soil for the plant to absorb.

Other factors contribute to magnesium deficiency. The way that we prepare foods removes magnesium. The process of boiling and steaming vegetables leaches magnesium into the water. Dietary phosphates found in soft drinks, high-sodium diets, high-sugar diets, excess insulin, diuretics, and other cardiac drugs all cause a loss of magnesium in the urine.

Good dietary sources of magnesium include dark green leafy vegetables, such as Swiss chard and spinach. The center of the chlorophyll molecule that gives green vegetables their color contains magnesium. Magnesium is also found in nuts and seeds, such as almonds, Brazil nuts, hazelnuts, pumpkin seeds, sesame seeds, and sunflower seeds.

Supplemental sources and dosages: A variety of magnesium supplements is on the market. Elemental magnesium, such as magnesium oxide, is the least expensive but also the least absorbable source. Chelated products such as magnesium glycinate or magnesium citrate are better options; they are more expensive but much more absorbable. Recommended dosages range from 400 to 1,000 mg daily.

Super Supplement #5: Multinutrient Formula

For general health purposes, a daily multivitamin is like a little added insurance. Unfortunately, even if you eat all the healthy foods recommended on the ancestral diet, you may not be getting all the nutrients you need to compensate for the depletion of nutrients in our soils, the abundance of environmental toxins that we deal with on a regular basis, and the chronic stress in our modern lives.

On page 83 is a list of what to look for in a multivitamin. The ingredients do not need to match this profile exactly, but you do want them to come close. One caveat is that you want to avoid iron unless you are a menstruating woman or a vegetarian. A number of studies suggest that too much of this mineral can increase your risk for heart disease and certain cancers.

Super Supplement #6: Glucosamine

It is not uncommon for clients over forty-five years of age to come in for training and have signs of osteoarthritis (OA), a degenerative disease of the joints. OA occurs when cartilage around your bones breaks down and is lost. Cartilage is the shock absorber between the bones of your joint; it protects your joints from damage when you are running, jumping, and performing other high impact movements.

Damage to your cartilage can occur through wear and tear over time from activities such as long-distance running or many years of playing soccer, especially when combined with an inflammatory high-carb diet. Or it can occur from trauma to the joint from playing physical contact sports, such as football or basketball.

Multinutrient Formula Ingredients

NUTRIENT	AMOUNT	NUTRIENT	AMOUNT
Vitamin A (as beta-carotene)	5,000 IU	Pantothenic acid	300 mg
Vitamin C	500–1,000 mg	Calcium	400 mg
Vitamin D	500–800 IU	Magnesium	400 mg
Vitamin E (as mixed tocopherols)	400 IU	Iodine	50 mcg
Vitamin B_1 (thiamine)	50 mg	Zinc	20 mg
Vitamin B_2 (riboflavin)	15 mg	Copper	2 mg
Vitamin B_3 (niacin)	30 mg	Selenium	100 mcg
Vitamin B6	20 mg	Manganese	3 mg
Folic acid	800 mcg	Chromium	250 mcg
Vitamin B_{12}	500–1,000 mcg	Molybdenum	100 mcg
(as methylcobalamin)		Boron	2 mg

Obesity and sedentary living are also risk factors, as cartilage requires movement for lubrication. And being overweight for a length of time with little muscle to support the joint, puts a great deal of stress on it.

One thing to keep in mind is that cartilage does not repair easily because it is predominantly avascular (without blood vessels). The compression and decompression of the surrounding tissue circulates the fluid that nourishes the cartilage. So, if you perform weight bearing or resistance exercise, you can get nourishment to the joint. *No movement, no nourishment.*

Once the joint is damaged, the immune system kicks in with the inflammatory response, and the joint becomes painful, inflamed, and swollen. This is where glucosamine sulfate comes in. Glucosamine is a naturally occurring amino sugar in the body that can also be synthesized from the amino acid L-glutamine and glucose.

Research suggests that supplemental glucosamine stimulates the production of cartilage-building proteins and inhibits the production of cartilage-destroying enzymes. It also reduces the symptoms of joint dysfunction—the pain, swelling, and tenderness—and improves overall mobility. Most people start to notice a difference after taking glucosamine for four weeks, but maximum benefits usually occur at eight to twelve weeks.

In the Primal Body Program, supplementing with glucosamine is combined with the ancestral diet to reduce inflammation, functional strength-training exercises to build muscle to support the joint, and stretching and foam rolling to improve the quality of the tissue and create overall structural integrity. Amazingly, many clients who come to me with joint pain, diagnosed as OA, are thrilled to find that they become pain free when they follow these simple steps.

Supplemental source and dosage: There are no major food sources of glucosamine, so supplementing is the only way to get it. Recommended dosages range from 1,500 to 3,000 mg daily.

Adding these supplements may seem like a lot, but it's for your body's greatest benefit. In Chapter 9, I'll give you suggestions for managing your supplements, so you can take them throughout the day.

While everyone may not need glucosamine, supplementing is a vital part of the Primal Body Program, one I urge all my clients to do.

Jennifer's Transformation
Reversing the Trend

In her own words, my client JENNIFER tells how the program helped her turn her life around, from heading in the direction of high medical bills for age-related illness to heading for the gym with a good attitude!

When I first started with the Primal Body Program six months ago, I was overweight, had no energy, and was a bit of a couch potato. In my youth in England, I had been very sporty and fit—played tennis, squash, field hockey, lacrosse, and cricket—but I gave all of it up when I started to work at eighteen. Therefore, at sixty-five years old, my muscles were nonexistent (I didn't have children to lift up and run after!). Consequently, not much energy! I really missed the "good old life" of sports and lots of energy, so I wanted to get back to my old self again.

PHEW! What hard work it was in the beginning! Yes, it hurt, and I rarely looked forward to going to the gym. I could NEVER have put myself through that pain and discomfort two or three times a week, but I trusted the program and that I would come to no harm. If I hurt somewhere or pulled a muscle (which usually meant that

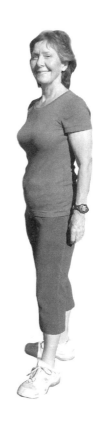

I hadn't been stretching enough), Mikki would know exactly what the remedy should be.

After six months of the gym, and having lost 20 pounds, I have learned exercise "etiquette" (don't complain as much!) and LOVE it when people notice that I have lost weight and look so good. My clothes are two sizes smaller—I gave my large clothes to Goodwill—and much more comfortable to wear.

My goal is to lose at least another 10 pounds (maybe 15) and still work on my muscle and body shape. It is easier going to the gym now. I look forward to the loss of each pound. Of course as well as providing weight training, stretching, and exercises, Mikki also tutored me on my eating habits (which were appalling, as I loved all the worst things!) and that has been a big contribution to my weight loss. Eating has been one of the most enjoyable activities in my life, so now I am learning to focus on other things to enjoy. Now I "eat to live" instead of "live to eat"!

Working with the Primal Body Program has turned my life around, helping me feel better about myself, I have more energy to accomplish more in my life, and I have more FUN! The investment has certainly paid off, and in the long run saves me from large medical bills in the future.

NEXT . . .

When you switch to the Primal Diet, you reduce the inflammation in your body and become less sedentary. As a result, fat begins to melt away. You will naturally begin to feel more energetic and have the kind of boundless energy our ancestors had when their survival depended on having a lean, fit, and healthy body.

Step 3: Restore Your Muscles to Pain-Free Movement shows you how to remove the adhesions and restrictions in your muscles resulting from sedentary living and injuries, so you can do the most congruent types of exercise for your human genome. A simple tool, the foam roller, helps you prepare for two kinds of Primal exercise: functional strength training (Step 4) and high-intensity interval training (Step 5).

Chapter 6

Step Three—Restore Your Muscles to Pain-Free Movement

Eating to get rid of painful inflammation is Step 1 in the Primal Body Program; increasing nutrient density through supplementation is Step 2; and restoring your muscles, tendons, ligaments, and fascia to pain-free movement is Step 3. These steps go hand in hand, supporting you to be able to move and exercise in a way that expresses your Primal physiologic inheritance. Although different people will need different amounts of restorative activity, almost everyone needs to attend to pain levels that restrict movement, before beginning the muscle building and metabolic interval training I recommend in Steps 4 and 5.

A pain-free body is a body ready and eager to exercise, allowing you to burn fat with speed and efficiency. You can restore your muscles to the condition best expressed by your genes using two techniques I show you in this chapter: (1) Self-Myofascial Release (SMR) with the foam roller, to reduce scar tissue and adhesions, decrease the density and overactivity of tight muscles, and improve mobility and range of motion; and (2) stretching, both passive and active, to lengthen muscles and surrounding tissue, for improved quality of movement.

Done together, these two techniques prepare you to take on Steps 4 and 5, which are the heart of your Primal Body training and exercise program. Not only will you be able to move with more ease and mobility, but you will also be preventing painful injuries that might result from tight muscles.

THE MESSAGE OF PAIN

One of the most common reasons people stop making progress in an exercise program and fall short of their fitness goals is pain caused by muscle tightness. In the Primal Body Program, instead of letting pain stop you, you pay attention to pain, learning how to release the muscle tightness causing that pain, so you can be pain free to move and exercise.

Often when I'm initially training people, they experience pain in their hip or knee on attempting simple movements, such as stepping up on a bench. This situation is more common than one would imagine. Hip pain, knee pain, back pain—all of these show up when the body is put under load for the first time, as is inevitable when you decide to become fit.

Dealing with pain is essential in any program that aims to help people who've been sedentary to get fit and lose weight. Pain on exercising is often a message from your body telling you about the condition of your muscles. The pain that shows up when you start to exercise is saying, "You need to release, lengthen, and strengthen your muscles."

THE COST OF SEDENTARY LIFESTYLES

Our ancient genes call for us to be physically active so as to maintain our health and fitness, but today, a sedentary lifestyle is more the norm. For us modern humans, the condition of our muscles is weak and stiff, due to sedentism and stress; and the tissue surrounding our muscles, the fascia, is tight and restrictive. This makes it difficult to move with ease, and as a result, injury to the muscle and tissue is a common event, whether it shows up as small tears or major disruptions that require lengthy recovery.

Of one thing we can be sure: When our cave-ancestors needed to make a quick getaway over a hill and through the brush, because a saber-toothed tiger was hot on their heels, they were not held back by muscle adhesions and chronic inflammation. If they had been, they would have been lunch and never survived to pass their genes down to us. In fact, because of their diet and activity patterns, our ancestors were much less likely to experience the kind of pain on movement or exertion we experience.

Unfortunately, we have adapted to the sedentism of our times by developing restriction in our muscles and in the fascial tissue that surrounds them, by means of bad postural habits and lack of use. A chronic tension keeps our muscles tight, and over time they are unable to perform even simple functions, such as holding the body upright in good posture and maintaining structural integrity of the body. You can see examples of this failure in the rounded shoulders of people who spend much of their time at a computer, or in the painful lower back of people carrying excess body weight.

Many of the aches and pains that people complain about as they get older are the result of dysfunctional postures and movements that lead to knots, dense tissue, and especially adhesions in the soft tissues of the body, making it painful to exert any force (as is needed when performing strength-building exercises). The overall effect is to restrict movement, causing even more tightness and dysfunction, a vicious cycle that results in a more sedentary lifestyle, which indirectly caused the problem in the first place.

HOW ADHESIONS FORM

Anyone who has ever torn or hurt a muscle has adhesions, which occur when the body tries to repair the damage caused by an injury. As part of the inflammatory and healing process, the body initiates mechanisms that attempt to regenerate the damaged tissue. This is not a perfect process. Usually, a less specialized tissue or form of collagen is produced in the process, not replicating exactly what was there before. Then the motion of the injured tissue influences the structure that forms when the tissue is healed.

If the limb does not get adequate movement while healing, it adheres to other muscle fibers, tendons, ligaments, or bones. This causes that part of the body to become nonfunctional and sometimes painful. Hence, you experience pain in your knee when you do that first step-up or lunge, and because of the discomfort, you don't want to continue. Your program gets stalled and eventually derailed, while you wait to heal.

The following exercise program is the way to restore your body back to a pain-free condition that leads to health, mobility, and flexibility.

THE SELF-MYOFASCIAL RELEASE TECHNIQUE

You can release chronic muscular tension by a technique known as Self-Myofascial Release (SMR). A simple tool that is becoming a staple in training programs worldwide, regardless of fitness level, is the foam roller. I will show you how to use the foam roller to release tightness and get rid of pain-causing adhesions in twelve different movements, but first let me explain what SMR is and how it works.

In Self-Myofascial Release, *myo* refers to muscle and *fascia* refers to the connective tissue that surrounds the muscle fibers. A more traditional way to release tightness in these tissues is through deep tissue massage, but using a foam roller is both more convenient and less expensive.

The way SMR works is that when you put pressure on a tight, tender area of the muscle, tiny sensing mechanisms located at the muscle-tendon junction are activated. When pressed, these sensors, called golgi tendon organs (GTO) stimulate the muscle spindles to relax the muscle in question, helping adhesions to release, blood flow to increase to the area, and the quality of the tissue to improve.

The SMR technique involves finding the painful spot and putting pressure on the area, using a tool such as the foam roller, for 1 or 2 minutes. During this time, you are consciously relaxing the area and releasing the knot, adhesion, or dense tissue. This takes focus and patience, especially if you have many painful spots and have not been stretching or doing activities to keep your muscles relaxed and elongated. But you'll notice that your efforts quickly pay off in the range of motion available immediately following an SMR session. And though it may be difficult in the beginning, once you learn the technique, it soon becomes a quick and easy way to release problems in the muscles and fascia.

FOAM ROLLER USE AND TECHNIQUE

The foam roller is a tool for doing SMR. With it, you can get near instant results by releasing chronic tension in the soft tissues (the muscles and the fascia that encapsulates them) and realigning the skeletal system in a way that makes it work better. More ease in your activities leads to greater ability to build muscle and burn fat through the kind of functional strength training and interval training I will show you how to do in Steps 4 and 5.

Also, when you begin to feel better in your body, you will want to do more playful activities, such as going for a walk on the beach or taking a dance class, both of which help improve fat loss and fitness, while not being perceived as work. Soon, you have changed from someone stuck in a sedentary existence to someone who is out and moving every day, reaping many of the benefits our ancestors had from their highly active lifestyle.

You can purchase a foam roller at most local sporting goods stores as well as online. But buyer beware: All foam rollers are not created equal. The white low-density rollers tend to lose their shape and break down easily. I recommend the black high-density rollers, which are firm and hold their shape well. I also recommend the Grid, a foam roller that is small enough to fit in a suitcase for travel. It has PVC underneath with softer material on top, giving it a nice firm feel. (See page 203 for more information.)

STEP 3

Nancy's Transformation
Pain-free Muscles Led
to Weight Loss

NANCY is a freelance editor and college instructor who's been working with me for seven months, starting her fitness program at age sixty-four. Initially, she dealt with painful adhesions in her muscles that severely restricted her ability to do the exercises I was prescribing. The foam roller was a major tool in her program to prepare her muscles for more rigorous training. In her own words:

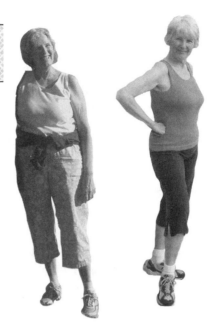

It was around my birthday that I was finally ready to get serious about my weight and health issues. I was about 20 pounds overweight, not sleeping well, and having injuries from falls. So at sixty-four, I told myself, I'm going to work with someone, since obviously I can't do it by myself. I met Mikki and thought, here is an experienced woman who isn't thirty years younger than me and who looks great, and that gave me hope.

I weighed 159 and was having trouble getting in and out of my car—not because of excess weight, but because I had such weak muscles and joints to move my weight. I'd park my car, open the door, and notice, GOSH IT'S TAKING ME A LONG TIME TO GET OUT OF THIS THING! WHEN DID THAT HAPPEN? I live in an upstairs condo and more and more I was asking my husband, "Honey, will you get these grocery bags?" He's a kind man so he did, but it was a sign to me that I was obviously deteriorating and needed to do something soon, or I'd lose my window.

I was worried that maybe I really needed a physical therapist, but Mikki was confident and said she could help me. I'd had a foot injury from falling the year before and had gone to a physical therapist for sessions that didn't help much. I'd also had sciatica in my left hip and lower back that had immobilized

me for a week. I had no muscle ability, very little strength! And I thought I CAN'T DO ANY OF THIS!

I learned from Mikki about something called functional training, which is amazing because you do exercises that translate to your everyday movements, for instance, getting in and out of your car. That's a hinging movement, I learned, bending from the hips and knees while keeping my back flat—a movement that is used frequently both in and out of the gym.

I could immediately apply what she was teaching me to my everyday activities, and so I started to get stronger right away. It was natural, even automatic to be developing strength by just doing what I did, and then I could exercise more and burn fat to lose that weight. Also, by doing the Primal movements, such as squats, I was reeducating myself on how to move. I also strengthened my core muscles, which I hadn't used in a while—I've been sitting in front of the computer for a few decades and had become very sedentary.

I was introduced to the foam roller for several of my issues. The first time I used it was because I couldn't do simple lunges without having knee pain. I could only do one or two and that was it. Mikki showed me how to use the foam roller on my quadriceps, and after a minute or two on each leg, I got back up and immediately could do a series of lunges. Now I do fifteen easily, in three repeated sets.

Previous to beginning my program, I had started to develop plantar fasciitis, a painful condition of the foot. I tried the self-myofascial release technique with a baseball and it went away very quickly. After a few months of using SMR and building strength, I was ready for a family hiking trip in Yellowstone. I used a foam roller on the arch of my foot every day, and was able to get up with ease and hike around without pain. Returning home, I started to jog and was able to do many activities of everyday life.

I still had adhesions and scar tissue from an old frozen shoulder injury; they were restricting my arm's full range of movement, and the muscle had atrophied somewhat. I thought I wouldn't be able to do the strength training because of how weak my muscles were. The foam roller was great for working all that out, and now I can do upper body exercises, like inverted rows and push-ups that I couldn't do before.

I jog for twenty minutes around my neighborhood every day now, and I work out three to four times a week, including going up and down stadium steps. My husband is inspired by my newfound fitness and often accompanies me on my jaunts and gym trips. It's easy and fun to do things that before were boring tasks—so boring I'd skip them! I also take a yoga or dance class once a week, or just go to my club for stretching and the treadmill.

I lost 17 pounds and feel so much more like myself now. Keeping a food journal and learning to eat the Primal way helped me drop the weight and also reduced the inflammation in my joints—a nice complement to using the foam roller. I'm now down to size 10 from 14, getting a big boost in how I feel about myself. I have more energy and don't ask my husband to carry the groceries upstairs for me anymore. I'm getting in and out of cars with ease, hinging before lowering my butt onto the seat, and getting out with a new bounce.

No more "little old lady" movements for me! I'm more mobile, more youthful, and so much more pain free following this program—a big benefit I never thought I'd get when I started out with weight loss as my goal.

SMR FOAM ROLLER EXERCISES

You can learn to use the foam roller on your own. However, a trainer can be invaluable when you are learning to use this new tool, as it can be uncomfortable at first and you can benefit by expert advice. (For more on choosing a trainer, see page 200.)

When I work with a client on using the foam roller, I assess which bodily areas would benefit from application by observing how the person moves in the seven Primal movement patterns—squat, lunge, push, pull, bend, twist, and gait (to be introduced in more detail in Step 4).

If you are *not* working with a trainer, pain can be your guide, showing you the areas of your body you need to roll out to adjust the tone and flexibility of your musculature. If after using the foam roller on your painful areas, function is restored and you can do the movement you couldn't do before, then you can assume you have released the problem. This is a process of experimentation, but over time, you will know exactly which areas benefit from doing the SMR technique with the foam roller.

12 SMR Foam Roller Exercises
EQUIPMENT: FOAM ROLLER, TENNIS BALL

Following is a list of muscle areas that may be tight and/or adhered, and suggested ways to use the foam roller for releasing them. For each of the foam roller exercises, roll slowly through the particular area until you find the tightest spot. Some areas will require more time than others, depending on the quality of the tissue, but spend at least a minute or two on each area in the beginning.

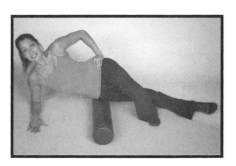

1. GLUTEUS MEDIUS

Lie on your side with the upper lateral area of the gluteal muscle resting on the foam roller. Place your same-side elbow and foot on the ground. Roll the entire muscle and stop on any sore spots. Switch sides and repeat.

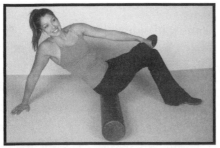

2. PIRIFORMIS

Sit on the foam roller, cross your right ankle over your left thigh, and lean into the meaty part of your right gluteal muscle while putting your left hand on your right ankle. Roll around this area and see if you can find any hot spots. Switch sides and repeat.

3. QUAD

Lie facedown with your upper body supported on your forearms and one thigh resting on the foam roller. Roll from your hip down to the top of the knee and lean from one side to the other to get to all four muscles. Switch legs and repeat.

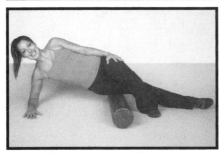

4. IT BAND

Lie on your right side with your body supported on your right elbow, the roller positioned just below your right hip, and your right leg fully extended. Bend the knee of your left leg and place the sole of your left foot on the floor in front of your right knee. Roll down the outside of your right leg until you reach the knee area. Switch legs and repeat.

5. ADDUCTOR

Lie facedown with your upper body supported on your forearms and the top of one inner thigh resting on the foam roller. Roll from your upper inner thigh down to just above the knee. Switch legs and repeat.

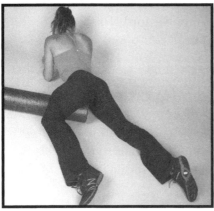

STEP 3

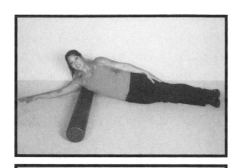

6. LAT

Lie on your right side with your right arm overhead, the foam roller under your armpit, and your body in a straight line. Roll from your armpit toward your hip, along the lat muscle. Switch sides and repeat.

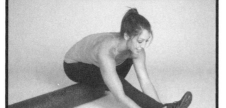

7. HAMSTRING

Sit up on the foam roller with the back of your right leg resting on the foam roller and your left foot positioned in alignment with the foam roller, sole on the floor. Lean forward with your upper body and roll from your hip down to your knee. You'll want to rotate your leg from side to side to reach all of the hamstring muscles. Switch legs and repeat.

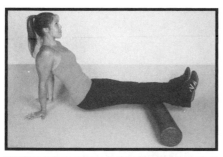

8. CALF

Balance on your hands with your lower legs resting on the foam roller. Roll from your ankle to your knee with your toes pointing toward you (dorsiflexion) and then pointing away (plantarflexion). To increase the intensity, stack one leg on top of the other.

9. PERONEAL

Lie on your right side with your upper body supported on your right elbow, legs extended, roller positioned just below your right knee. Roll down the lateral area of your lower right leg. Switch legs and repeat.

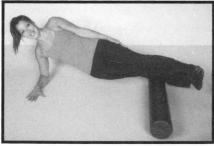

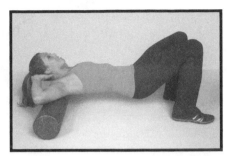

10. UPPER BACK

Lie back with your arms behind your head and the roller positioned beneath your upper back. With your elbows pointing out, roll your upper back/shoulder blade area. Roll to the left or right to emphasize one side or the other.

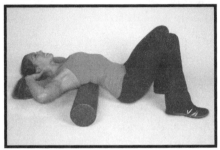

11. MIDBACK

Lie back with the foam roller positioned under your midback. With your hips raised, roll from the base of your shoulder blades to the top of the pelvis, emphasizing one side and then the other.

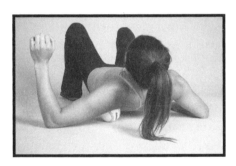

12. ROTATOR CUFF

Lie on your back with a tennis ball or larger softball placed between your upper arm and shoulder blade and the floor. Place your upper arm on the floor and bend your elbow to 90 degrees. Slowly internally and externally rotate your shoulder by moving your hand back and forth with your elbow bent.

STRETCHING TO BECOME PAIN FREE

A comprehensive approach to becoming pain free, as well as preventing future pain from possible injury, includes following the foam roller with a series of passive stretches. First roll, then stretch. Both approaches correct sedentary living effects and can help restore movement capacity, preparing you for the functional training that follows in the next two steps. With movement restored, staying fit and keeping weight off is natural and easy.

I will show you two ways to stretch and improve the health of your muscles: static stretching for flexibility and active stretching for mobility. Stretching for flexibility should follow your foam roller sessions, whereas stretching for mobility increases the range of motion of your joints and can be used as a warm-up for your training.

STATIC STRETCHING FOR FLEXIBILITY

The foam roller and static stretching go hand in hand; the roller helps you remove restrictions, and then static stretching helps you restore muscle to its proper length. Because restrictions are removed, the muscle is ready to be stretched after foam rolling.

Imagine a rubber band that has a knot tied in it. If you try to stretch a rubber band that has a knot in it, the band will most likely break at the point where the knot is. Once the knot is removed, however, you can stretch the band without causing a break. Muscles are like rubber bands; knots in them are likely to cause tears and stop lengthening, so getting the knots out first with the foam roller allows muscles to elongate on stretching.

Flexibility is defined as the measure of a joint's movement through a normal range of motion. A flexible joint has the ability to move through a greater range of motion, so you're much less likely to become injured in the course of your everyday activities and sports if you stretch for joint flexibility.

Flexibility training for improving posture and reducing pain involves lengthening a muscle through static stretching. Poor postural habits can cause your muscles and the connective tissue that surrounds them to shorten and mold into the positions you maintain throughout your day (such as the rounded shoulders that develop from spending too many hours in front of a computer). Stretching these short, tight muscles helps lengthen the muscle, which then allows the body to realign the soft tissue structures, so it's a lot easier to maintain good posture.

Probably the greatest benefit is the effect stretching has on the lower back. By increasing the flexibility of your hamstrings, hip flexors, quadriceps, and other muscles that attach to the pelvis, you reduce the tension on the lumbar spine, so you're much less prone to suffer from low back pain.

One more point of interest is that researchers claim stretching immediately before exercise does *not* prevent injury, and it may actually make you weaker. Stretching after training, however, is effective to reduce muscle soreness. So stretch following your workouts, when your muscles are warmed up for the maximum benefit.

STRETCHES TO INCREASE FLEXIBILITY

EQUIPMENT: MAT OR TOWEL; STABILITY BALL (BE SURE TO USE A BALL THAT IS ANTI-BURST, WHICH MEANS THAT THE BALL WILL DEFLATE SLOWLY IF IT IS PUNCTURED WHILE YOU ARE ON IT; IT WILL NOT SUDDENLY COLLAPSE UNDER YOU.)

For each stretch, focus on the muscle you want to stretch and gently move your body into the position, until you have reached the desired level of tension (accompanied by a feeling of discomfort but not pain) in the muscle. Hold the position for 30 to 60 seconds, then release. Never bounce or jerk while stretching. Relax your breathing and visualize your muscles, tendons, and ligaments all lengthening as you stretch.

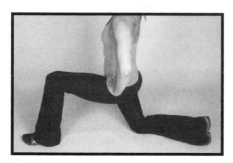

1. HIP FLEXOR STRETCH

Lunge forward with one knee on a mat and the other foot flat on the floor. Squeeze your glutes and straighten the hip above your back leg by pushing your hips forward. Relax and repeat with the other side.

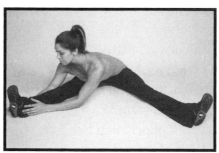

2. HAMSTRING STRETCH

Sit on a mat with your legs pointing to the diagonal and knees extended. Bring your chest toward one leg while keeping the knee extended. Relax and repeat with the other leg.

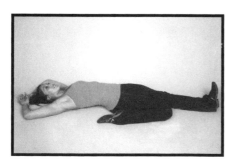

3. QUAD STRETCH

While sitting on a mat, bend one knee behind you and lower yourself back until you are resting on your elbows. Continue, if possible, until your back is on the floor. Relax and repeat with the other leg.

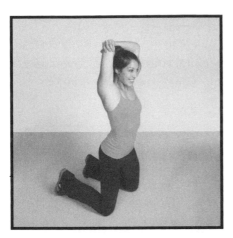

4. TRICEP STRETCH

Standing, kneeling, or sitting, grasp one elbow overhead with your opposite hand. Pull your elbow back and toward your head. Relax and repeat with the other arm.

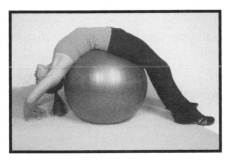

5. ABDOMINAL STABILITY BALL STRETCH

Start by sitting on a stability ball and lower yourself down until the middle of your back is resting on the ball. Gently lean back, with your arms overhead, and extend your arms and legs until they reach the floor, if possible.

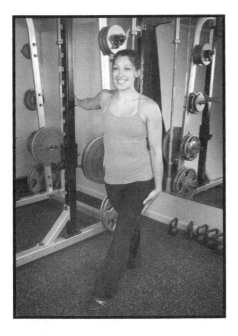

6. PEC STRETCH

With your arm extended, position your hand on a doorway or structure at shoulder height. Turn your body away from your arm to stretch. Relax and hold stretch. Repeat with opposite arm.

Note: Your upper chest becomes more stretched with the elbow lower; your lower chest becomes more stretched with elbow the higher.

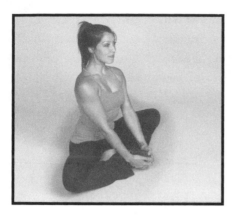

7. ADDUCTOR STRETCH

Sit on a mat. Bring the soles of your feet together and pull your feet toward your groin. Press your knees toward the floor.

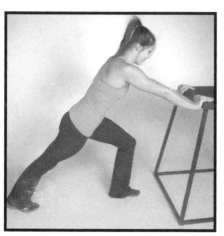

8. CALF STRETCH

Place both hands on a wall or stable surface and extend your arms. Lean into the surface with one leg bent forward and the other leg extended back. Push the heel of the back leg down to execute the stretch.

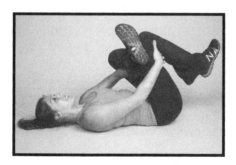

9. HIP STRETCH

Lie back on a mat. Cross the ankle of one leg over the thigh of the other leg. Grasp the hamstring of the leg that has the ankle crossed over it with both hands and pull your leg toward your chest until you feel the stretch in your buttocks. Relax and repeat with the other leg.

STEP 3

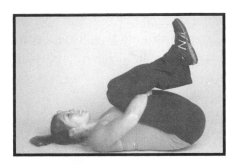

10. LOW BACK STRETCH

Lie back on a mat with your head on the floor. Bend both of your knees and grasp the back of your thighs behind your knees. Pull your knees toward your shoulders and hold.

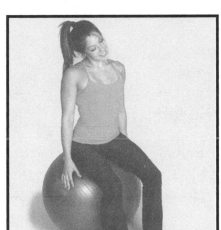

11. NECK STRETCHES (ALL THREE PLANES OF MOTION)

SIDE TO SIDE

Sit on a mat or stability ball. Bend your neck and bring your ear close to your shoulder, relax, drop your shoulders, and hold. Repeat on the other side.

FRONT TO BACK

Sit on a mat or stability ball. Bring your chin toward the top of your chest, relax, drop your shoulders, and hold. Then move your chin away from your chest, relax, drop your shoulders, and hold.

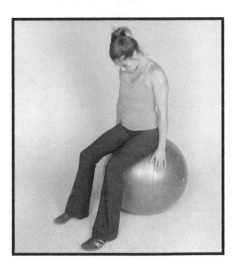

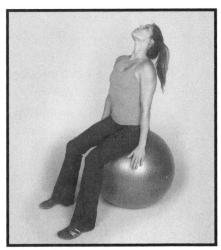

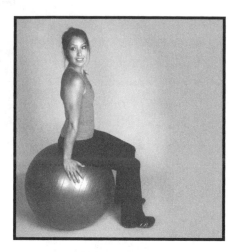

ROTATION

Sit on a mat or stability ball. Rotate your face toward one shoulder, relax, drop your shoulders, and hold. Repeat on the other side.

ACTIVE STRETCHING FOR MOBILITY

Whereas flexibility is the ability to move joints freely through a full range of motion, mobility is the ability to move joints through a full range of motion with control. Contrasted to flexibility, mobility involves active movement and requires strength to produce a joint's full range of motion.

Many individuals prepare for their training by performing static stretches prior to their workout. However, though stretching helps to improve (nonmoving) flexibility, it may not do such a good job at preparing your body to move quickly and efficiently. That's why I recommend mobility exercises to loosen up before working out or competing in sports. Dynamic mobility exercises prepare your body for the vigorous movements that make up the more demanding part of your training or sports.

Joint mobility exercises work by circulating the synovial fluid (lubricant) that washes the joints. Because joints have no direct blood supply, this fluid provides nutrition and simultaneously removes waste products. When performed correctly, joint mobility exercises can restore complete range of motion to the ankles, knees, hips, shoulders, spine, neck, elbows, wrists, and fingers.

Use mobility exercises as your warm-up and perform static stretches after the workout or sports competition as part of the cooldown to restore tissue length and prevent long-term injury. Static exercises help bring the body back to a state of rest and recovery and allow you to focus on relaxing and lengthening the muscles that you just put under stress while you were exercising or playing sports.

Mobility Drills

The following mobility drills are dynamic exercises that prepare you for activity. These movements increase the blood flow to your muscles, increasing your range of motion and your body temperature, and they stimulate your nervous system, so your mind and body are ready to go. Begin with a series of joint rotations, and then perform several jumping jacks, or alternate drills to vary the routine.

JOINT ROTATIONS

Start in a standing position with your arms hanging at your sides. Then rotate each of the following joints slowly in both directions, about eight times in each direction.

1. Neck
2. Shoulders
3. Elbows
4. Wrists
5. Hips
6. Knees
7. Ankles

JUMPING JACKS

This is the old-fashioned exercise that baby boomers will recall from many years ago. Stand with your feet together and arms at your sides. Jump up, moving your feet apart and raising your arms over your head. Jump again and bring your feet together and your arms back to your sides. Perform 20 repetitions, then rest.

NEXT . . .

Once you have learned how to roll out painful adhesions with the foam roller and begun stretching to gain mobility and flexibility, you are ready for the next step in the Primal Body Program: building muscle strength through functional training.

Functional training teaches you how to use your body for everyday fitness, whether you are an athlete, a weight-loss candidate, or just someone who wants to stay fit using the best possible technique. Functional training relies on the seven Primal movements that you will learn about in Step 4, which best express your genetic inheritance and can be done at any age. It is your fastest route to having a lean and muscular body, because it mimics your 2-million-year-old genetic blueprint.

Chapter 7

Step Four—Build Muscle with Primal Movement

The first three steps of the Primal Body Program showed you how to reduce inflammation through diet and supplementation, and release restrictions in your muscles, leaving you pain-free and ready to move. Now, in Step 4, I show you how to exercise your body and build muscle as our early human ancestors did, so you can restore your body's inherited ability to move with grace and power.

The Primal Body Program assumes that we are all natural-born athletes, fully equipped with everything we need to rapidly and effectively respond to a variety of physical challenges. The problem is that modern bodies don't get many physical challenges, partly due to conveniences brought about by the agricultural revolution. We don't have the daily challenge of hunting game for food, fleeing from predators, or hoisting heavy tree trunks into place for our shelter. Through sedentary living, we've lost touch with the basic patterns of Primal movement, and so developed muscle imbalances and asymmetries, leading to faulty movement patterns, and, in some cases, overall dysfunction.

In Step 4, I introduce functional strength training, an approach to fitness that emphasizes full-body movements rather than isolated muscle movements done on machines. Functional strength training is the first part of this training program. Then, in Step 5, you will learn the second part, metabolic training (also referred to as cardiovascular training), using high-intensity interval training (HIIT) interspersed with low-intensity "play" activities, such as swimming, hiking, and walking.

Together, functional strength training and metabolic training provide the closest approximation of exercise to your genetic blueprint, allowing you to take advantage of your physiology as it was designed to be lean, fit, and healthy. As you continue in the Primal Body Program, I will show you how to bring the two approaches together into a unique hybrid training that is highly effective for both building muscle and burning fat. Then in Chapter 10, you will see how to put it all together in a customized program for your individual use. Keep in mind that while the material in this chapter and the next may seem like a lot all at once, you will be able to use it in a plan I will help you design.

FUNCTIONAL TRAINING

When I started out as a personal trainer twenty years ago, people who came to me were in better shape than are the people I see today. Today, people are starting out in much worse condition, due to an increase in sedentary lifestyles.

On top of that, people eat more fast foods and have more stress, both of which show up in their body, often as more body fat and less muscle. All of these changes affect their ability (or lack of ability) to perform basic movements, many of which are Primal movements that our ancestors performed, such as simple squats or step-ups.

As a result of this trend, many personal trainers have completely overhauled their approach to training. Before the trend, an exercise program typically involved a body-building type of workout. Exercises were grouped by body parts, the individual working different parts of the body on different days of the week. One such routine might be chest and back on Monday, legs on Wednesday, and shoulders and arms on Friday. Low-intensity aerobic exercise was performed on the days of the week one was not lifting weights, and stretching was recommended. But all that is changing.

Functional training departs from more traditional workout programs by shifting the focus to full body exercise, no longer focusing on isolating body parts to build muscle. Instead, the goal of functional exercise is to restore function by uncovering muscle imbalances and faulty movement patterns caused by weak links in the kinetic chain, and then correcting them.

The kinetic chain is a linkage system; it links adjacent joints and muscles together so that energy, or force, generated by one part of the body can move successfully through the body. When you have a weakness in one segment, the body tries to compensate by misusing other body parts. Once these weak links in the kinetic chain are corrected—by releasing restrictions using the foam roller and building strength and awareness with Primal/functional movement patterns—you will be able to move the way your body was designed to move.

Functional/Primal movement patterns not only correct these imbalances, but they will prepare you for the activities of your daily life. For example, a functional exercise such as stepping up on a bench with dumbbells in your hands and pressing the dumbbells overhead will prepare you to step up on a chair to put a box on a shelf. The idea is to work against the resistance in such a way that the strength gained from the exercise transfers to a specific movement in life. This is the essence of functional training.

Unlike the earlier, traditional approach of working one muscle at a time, as in body-building training, functional strength training involves combining exercises to get all the muscles working together. This is not only a more natural movement pattern that we use in everyday life, but it is the movement pattern that early hunter-gatherers used in their lives.

Coach Mike Boyle points to another aspect of functional training when he defines it in his book *Functional Training for Sports*: "Functional training is best described as a continuum of exercises that teaches athletes to handle their own body weight in all planes of movement."[1] He's pointing to the fact that we humans perform a wide range of movements (walking, running, pushing, pulling, bending, twisting, starting, stopping, etc.) that take place in all three planes—front to back, side to side, and rotational. Because of this, you should train in all three planes, not just the front-to-back plane emphasized in the traditional gym setting.

But at the very essence, functional training is about purpose. When you train this way, you are preparing yourself for the specific activities of your life. And some exercises are more functional than others.

In the traditional gym setting, for example, the machine leg curl has been considered a staple of lower-body strength training. It's an isolation exercise (a single joint movement) stressing knee flexion, used for strengthening the hamstrings. However, this exercise is useless, because you never use the muscle action of isolated knee flexion, (especially when lying on your stomach) in everyday activities and sports. The leg curl is nonfunctional, meaning there's no transfer to it.

In activities such as walking, running, and jumping, the function of the hamstrings is not to flex the knee but to extend the hip. So, to develop functional strength for these activities, you want to perform hip extension exercises where your foot is in contact with the ground. This is known as a closed-chain exercise, as opposed to an open-chain exercise where your foot, or the limb that's working, is not in contact with the ground, such as the leg curl.

In addition, your hamstrings don't work in isolation; rather, they work together with your glutes (buttocks) in almost all movements to create hip extension. So, an exercise such as the one-leg stiff-leg deadlift (demonstrated on page 124), which strengthens the glutes and hamstrings at the same time, is a great functional movement, because it works the muscles in ways that you actually use them in your everyday life and sports.

BENCH DIPS ON A SEAWALL

A client asked me recently for exercises to firm muscles on the back of her upper arms, the triceps. Summer was around the corner, and she wanted to go sleeveless without worrying about unsightly flabby upper arms.

Using my approach of functional training, I demonstrated in the gym how to perform bench dips, an exercise to strengthen the triceps muscles. My client repeated my movements, putting her hands behind her on a low bench, feet on the floor, and gradually lowering her body in front of the bench until her butt touched the floor. By doing this, she was using her triceps to lift and lower her entire body weight, an effective way to build muscle.

However, after one attempt at this exercise, she found it too difficult and asked whether I could show her an easier exercise to accomplish the same goal. It was the perfect opportunity to explain how functional training is a better approach than more traditional—and possibly easier—approaches. I explained how easier exercises for the triceps, such as dumbbell kickbacks—done while the knee, foot, and hand rest on a bench and you extend the elbow of your opposite arm—had little transfer value to movements done routinely in her daily life, and therefore were not as effective in building muscle. On the other hand, an exercise such as the bench dip, I further explained, relates directly to natural movements done in the course of her day and so will prepare her to do that movement better. The bonus is she'd be building muscle for use both in and out of the gym.

To further make the point, I suggested that she visit the Santa Barbara Harbor and walk out on the breakwater. There I suggested she attempt to lift herself up on the 3-foot-high concrete sea wall to sit and enjoy a relaxing view of the ocean. She balked, saying she'd probably never be able to lift her body weight up onto the wall. But after a few more sessions of doing bench dips in the gym, she took my advice and surprised herself by finding the 3-foot hop up easier to accomplish than she'd thought.

This is a perfect example of functional training, because the exercises are whole body and Primal. Once you learn to train functionally, you won't want to go back to isolating muscles and joints on machines to miss having your hard work translated into everyday results. Functional movement exercises prepare you for the

Principles of Functional Training

1. Functional training is purposeful; there's a reason for the exercises, which is to prepare you for movement in your daily life or sports.
2. Functional exercises train full-body movements, not individual muscles, without the use of machines.
3. Functional movements involve multiple joints in multiple planes, whereas more traditional single joint exercises isolate specific muscles, and are therefore not very useful.
4. Functional training incorporates balance and proprioception (internal sense of where you are in space) into the exercise program. Single-leg exercises are emphasized as a way to improve balance.
5. In MOST functional exercises (such as the pull-up), the foot or hand that is working is in contact with the ground or a stable surface. So, the chain is closed; an open chain is when the foot or hand that is working is not in contact with a stable surface (such as in the lat pull-down).

(Adapted from Mike Boyle's *Functional Training for Sports*)

activities of your life. In my client's case, lifting her body weight to a higher ground was the kind of movement our ancestors might have used to escape a predator or avoid drowning in a flash flood.

SEVEN PRIMAL MOVEMENT PATTERNS

Functional training, because it emphasizes full-body movements in all three planes and translates to common activities, is the essence of Primal movement—the closest you can come to moving as our early human ancestors did.

The link to Primal movement is even clearer when we see how functional training simulates the seven Primal movement patterns, distinct movements that our ancestors would have had to perform effortlessly to survive. Identified by physical therapist Paul Chek on his Web site,[2] these seven basic movements consist of squatting, lunging, bending, pushing, pulling, twisting, and gait (as detailed in the following chart) and would have been used in ancient activities, such as shooting a bow and arrow, hoisting a spear, or lifting a heavy rock. Failure of muscles to fire in any of these patterns would cause a momentary hesitation in, for example, an early hunter's attempt to bring down a large mammal, possibly costing him his life.

The 7 Primal Movements

Type of Movement	Directions	Exercise Examples	Primal Movement Examples
1. Squat	Bend knees and hips, keeping back straight and knees pointed in the same direction as feet, and descend until thighs are parallel to the floor. Return by extending knees and hips until legs are straight and you are standing.	Kettlebell squat, barbell squat, or prison squats	Squatting down to gather wild herbs and plants
2. Lunge	Step forward and lower knee of opposite leg until knee is almost in contact with the floor. Return by pushing off front foot and bringing both feet together.	Front lunges, lateral lunges, or reverse lunges	Lunging forward to throw a spear
3. Bend	Bend your hips and knees while pushing your hips back and keeping your back straight, also known as hinging. Return to standing by extending hips and knees, bringing your hips forward.	Kettlebell swings, barbell deadlifts, or one-leg stiff-leg deadlifts	Bending over to clear a rock to make camp
4. Push	Use your upper body to push a weight away from you, or to push yourself away from the ground or other stable surface.	Push-ups, one-arm stability ball chest press, or kettlebell military press	Pressing a log overhead to carry back to camp or catching yourself when you fall forward
5. Pull	Use your upper body to pull a weight toward you or to pull yourself toward a stable surface.	Inverted rows, or horizontal pull-ups, pull-ups, or prone rows	Pulling heavy game back to camp or pulling up on a tree branch to avoid danger
6. Twist	This movement is usually combined with other Primal movements, such as squatting or rowing, and involves rotating the torso.	Reverse medicine ball wood chop or T push-up	Throwing a spear or twisting to avoid a tree branch while hiking
7. Gait	Walk, jog, or sprint.	Walking, jogging, or sprinting	Sprinting to avoid a predator or walking to track wild game

These seven movements may already exist in one form or another in your exercise regimen. If they do, challenge yourself with the following variations, including using the kettlebell, a tool I give further instructions for using later in this chapter. If they don't exist for you, incorporate them in your routine for something new and different. To make this easier for you, in a following section, "Primal Body Foundation Exercises," I describe a set of fourteen exercises that incorporate the seven Primal movements presented here.

Kettlebells: The Ultimate Functional Training Tool

If you're not familiar with the kettlebell, this training tool looks like a cannonball with a handle. It's this shape that makes the kettlebell so different from using a dumbbell. The design causes the weight of the bell to hang off your body, creating an offset center of gravity. This causes your body to utilize core, stabilizing muscles to create balance.

Another difference is that the kettlebell creates momentum, because it swings. Dumbbells don't offer that. In daily life, we pick up grocery bags, we pick up kids and animals, and we move things around. These activities all have momentum. Training with kettlebells prepares us for these types of functional activities.

The kettlebell is a highly functional training tool; it effectively increases strength, power, speed, coordination, and core stability. The workouts are intense, and they cause your body to hit the kind of metabolic peaks our ancestors experienced in their movement patterns.

Incorporating kettlebell training into my own personal workouts has brought some surprising results. Amazingly, after years of advanced/heavy lifting, I discovered that as a result of kettlebell training with Pavel Tsatsouline (see page 45), I was actually getting in better shape.

Before I attended his seminar, I knew some trainers who had been to one of Pavel's previous seminars, and I joked about how they came back as Russian Kettlebell Challenge (RKC) clones. Another trainer commented that there must have been a chip implanted in their brain, because they came back so over the top in their enthusiasm about KB training. I swore the same thing would never happen to me.

But even with that intention, it still happened! I was and continue to be highly enthusiastic about kettlebell training, because after many years of performing free-weight exercises with great proficiency, I am now getting in better condition with kettlebells. This is because in the context of the SAID principle (see page 113), the challenge imposed by kettlebells is different and greater than what I had previously experienced, so my body is adapting.

And the science backs up my experience. A study done in 1983 by a Russian researcher named V. I. Voropayev validates just how effective kettlebell training can be. In this study, two groups of college students were followed over several years. One group used a standard military regimen of pull-ups, 100-meter sprints, standing broad jumps, and a 1 km run. The experimental group used nothing but kettlebells and kettlebell exercises.

After several years of training, both groups were tested, using the same traditional exercises as the standard military group. Amazingly, the kettlebell group scored higher in every test—even though they had never practiced those particular exercises!

KETTLEBELL WARNING

Kettlebell training is becoming increasingly widespread in gyms and with trainers. However, some trainers may be using poor technique and unsafe training practices.

Kettlebells can be unsafe if proper technique is not followed. I was trained and certified by Pavel Tsatsouline and my instructions for kettlebell use as shown in this book are in accordance with Pavel's teaching.

If you are interested in advanced training with kettlebells, make sure you are guided by a professional who is formally trained by the RKC, which requires a high level of fitness and excellent technique to pass the certification, or other reliable source.

I recommend that women purchase an RKC brand 8 kg (18-pound), 12 kg (26-pound), and 16 kg (35-pound) kettlebell and that men purchase a 12 kg (26-pound), 16 kg (35-pound), and 20 kg (44 pound) kettlebell. Please keep in mind that these are general guidelines. If you are super strong, you might want to pick up a heavier bell. Or, if you are out of shape, try something lighter. For information about where to purchase kettlebells, see page 203.

HOW TO GET RESULTS

If building muscle is your goal, there's one basic notion you'll want to adhere to. It's called progressive overload. The concept comes from the Greek legend about a wrestler named Milo who lived in the city-state of Crotona. According to the tale, Milo put a baby calf on his shoulders every day and walked around a large stadium. As the calf began to grow, Milo grew, too, developing the muscles he needed to carry the animal. Eventually, Milo became so strong that one day he was able to carry a full-grown bull on his shoulders.

This was the beginning of the concept of progressive overload, which states that you need to increase the demand you impose on your body if you want to continue to gain muscle. Whether your goal is to add muscle for better athletic performance or to turn that middle-aged flab into well-defined arms, butt, and abs, the demand, or load, you place on your body is what's going to get your body to change.

While you may not have access to a calf to carry or a stadium to circumnavigate, there are a number of ways you can bring the principle of progressive overload into your own regimen and use it to harness your body's physiology. I'm going to show you exactly how to load your body in a way that is progressive and natural, matching the original pressures of the environment your body evolved in response to, over millions of years. But first, some basic physiology so you can understand the design of your body and how to utilize the principles of its design for maximum results.

When designing a strength-building program, keep in mind that the human body is resistant to change; it wants to remain the same. This is what scientists refer to as homeostasis. Homeostasis is defined as the ability of the body to maintain a condition of equilibrium or stability within its internal environment, when dealing with external changes. An example is when your body regulates your internal temperature to stay around 98.6 degrees: We sweat to cool off during the hot summer months and shiver to produce heat during the cold winter season.

This same principle of homeostasis applies to body weight, body composition, and strength. For your body to change, you need to impose a demand that overloads it in a way that it is not accustomed to, so as to bring about a particular outcome.

Imposing a demand is guided by something called the SAID principle. SAID is an acronym which stands for "specific adaptation to imposed demand." It means that when your body is placed under some form of stress, it starts to make adaptations that will allow it to get better at withstanding that specific form of stress in the future. While there are innumerable mechanisms involved in the adaptation process, the general idea is that your body will get better at the specific thing you do.

For example, if you stress the bones of your body through repeated impact, your body will respond by hardening the bones in the area where they were stressed. The same thing happens to tendons and ligaments when they are subjected to repeated stress through resistance training, making them thick and strong. Similarly, repeated stress will cause muscles to get bigger and stronger. The bottom line is that unless you impose a demand greater than what your body is already capable of, your body will not change and you will not get stronger.

Here are my suggestions for incorporating progressive overload into your exercise regimen:

Use your own body weight. Begin with simple body-weight exercises, such as push-ups and squats. Once you have mastered these basic exercises and you can support your own body weight, progress by increasing the difficulty to more challenging body-weight exercises. For example, start with the split squat (rear foot on the floor), and progress to split squatting with your rear foot elevated on a bench. Then advance to the forward lunge, the walking lunge, and finally the lunge jump. When doing push-ups, start by supporting your weight on a bench rather than on the floor, and progress to the floor when you are stronger.

Add weights. Once you can support your own body weight, begin to add weight, or resistance, while keeping the number of repetitions the same. For example, while performing the split squat with rear foot elevated, do a set of 5 repetitions with 10 pounds (5-pound dumbbells in each hand). Then in the next workout, do a set of 5 reps with 20 pounds. Then in the following workout, do a set of 5 reps of the same exercise with 30 pounds.

Increase repetitions. Another method of progressive overload involves adding repetitions while keeping the weight the same. For example, in the first workout you do a set of 5 reps with 25 pounds. In the second, you do a set of 6 reps with 25 pounds. And in the third, you do a set of 7 reps with 25 pounds.

Increase volume. One more variation is to increase the training volume by adding more sets to the workout. For example, in one workout you perform 12 sets per workout. In the next workout you perform 13 sets. Then, in the following workout, you perform 14 sets per workout.

STABILIZING YOUR CORE

Early in the trend toward functional training, strength coaches and personal trainers started seeing a pattern of problems involving certain parts of the body that require stabilization: the hips, trunk, and posterior shoulder. Because these core areas were weak, they were repeatedly causing problems and injuries.

To avoid injury, therefore, it's recommended to add core exercises to your functional training, to strengthen your body's stabilizers. Although core exercises appear to be nonfunctional, not ground based, they are an important part of the functional training program. Strengthening these muscles corrects problems caused by sedentary living and returns function to the body.

One example of muscle imbalances caused by sedentary living is sitting in front of the computer. This posture causes rounded shoulders, because it encourages weak lower trapezius muscles in the upper back, and short, tight pectoralis/chest muscles. Likewise, long periods of sitting also cause the gluteal (butt) muscles to stop firing; they become elongated and dormant, while the antagonist hip flexors become short and tight. Because the glutes no longer fire properly, the hamstrings and lower back have to pick up more of the load, and the result is often low back pain. (The glute muscles are not stabilizers though; they are prime movers and should be strengthened with functional hip extension movements.)

Here's how it all works: A stabilizer is defined as a muscle that contracts with no significant movement to maintain a posture or fixate a joint. This type of muscle is not directly involved in moving a weight, for example. A stabilizer's job is to keep certain parts of the body still, so that the muscles directly involved in moving a weight—the prime movers—can work effectively.

Three key areas of the body that require stabilizing are the trunk, hips, and posterior shoulders. Here is the physiology involved in strengthening and stabilizing these three areas:

The trunk is stabilized primarily by the transversus abdominus and multifidus muscles. The transversus abdominus is the deepest layer of abdominal muscle that runs from the pubic bone to the upper rib cage and attaches to the spine via the lumbar fascia, The multifidus is located along the back of the spine. These muscle groups work together to stabilize or stiffen the core through a "bracing" technique. Most people with low back pain have dysfunction/weakness in these important muscles.

The hips require stabilization for movements such as walking, running, and single-leg exercises, such as the one-leg squat. The gluteus medius muscle is the main stabilizer of the hip joint, and strengthening this muscle helps prevent injuries to the knee as well as improving the power of the quadriceps.

The shoulder is the most mobile joint in the body, and it, too, requires stabilization for correct mechanics and injury prevention. The lower trapezius muscle stabilizes the shoulder blades during movement. Engaging these stabilizers, by seating the shoulder blades—pulling them down and back—can help prevent rotator cuff injuries. It also reduces upper trapezius activity, which is one of the main causes of neck pain and tension.

Strengthening the stabilizers is necessary, not only to avoid injury, but also because stronger stabilizers will affect the amount of weight you're able to lift while strength training. For example, in the kettlebell military press exercise (see page 125), the amount of weight you can lift is affected by the stabilizers of the trunk and shoulders. Regardless of your strength, if your stabilizers are weak, you won't be able to lift as much weight.

In addition to your doing specific core exercises, these stabilizers can be developed through functional training. Functional training, without the use of machines, requires that *you* be your own stabilizer. When you perform unilateral movements, such as one-leg squats and one-leg stiff-leg deadlifts, with good form, you develop the stabilizers of the hips, trunk, and shoulders. Holding your body tight, or bracing, while exercising is one of the best ways to do this.

According to Stuart McGill, the spinal mechanics expert, "Good technique in most sporting and daily living tasks demands that power be generated at the hips and transmitted through a stiffened core."

Here are the six core strengthening and stabilizing exercises I recommend to be incorporated in your functional strength-training regimen. (You'll see that I don't mention numbers of reps; remember, I'll show you in Chapter 10 how to put all this together for your own customized program.)

6 Core Exercises
EQUIPMENT: MAT, STABILITY BALL

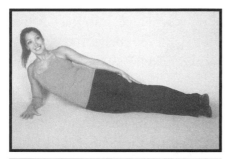

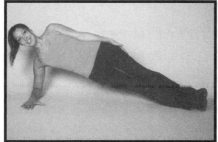

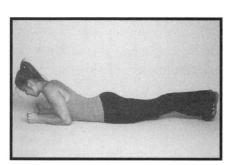

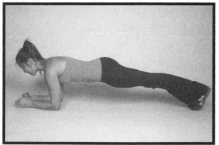

1. SIDE BRIDGE

This is a lateral flexion exercise for developing stability in the lumbar spine.

Action: Lie on your elbow with your top hip stacked above your bottom hip. Raise yourself up until your body is in a straight line through your feet, hips, and head. Lower your body down under control until your hips barely touch the ground. Repeat this sequence for the desired number of repetitions. Then switch to the other side and repeat.

Comments: This exercise should be done without using any rotation to get yourself up. Beginners might want to bend the knee of the bottom leg to 90 degrees to decrease the difficulty.

2. PRONE BRIDGE

This develops stunning core strength. There are three different levels to this exercise. I suggest working through the progression using the method outlined here.

Action: Lie facedown on the ground or floor and stretch out your limbs. Lift your body up so that you are balanced on your forearms and toes. Now tuck your pelvis under. This basically means rotating the lower part of your pelvis toward the ground, also referred to as posterior pelvic tilt. This tilt should cause you to go into a neutral spine, where there's almost no extension in the lumbar spine. Then hold this position for 30 seconds and rest.

To increase the difficulty of this exercise, get into the position where you are balanced on your forearms and toes with your pelvis tucked. Then raise one leg and hold for 30 seconds. Repeat on the other side for 30 seconds and then rest.

To advance this exercise one step further, once again, get into the position where you are balanced on your forearms and toes with your pelvis tucked. Then raise your opposite arm and leg simultaneously and hold for 30 seconds. Repeat on the other side for 30 seconds and then rest.

Comments: This exercise not only develops strength in the muscles involved, it also teaches you to maintain stability (relative stillness) in the lumbar spine while performing exercises in the prone position, such as push-ups and prone rows.

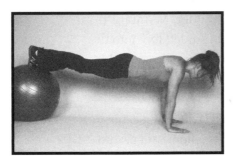

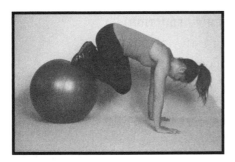

3. STABILITY BALL JACKKNIFE
This targets your lower abdominals. Because the ball is unstable, your entire core has to work to maintain the position of your body.

Action: Start by getting into a push-up position with the tops of your feet on a stability ball. Your body should form a straight line from your toes to your shoulders, with your hands positioned just slightly wider than your shoulders.

Keeping your back flat and abs tight, bend your knees and hips and roll the ball toward your torso. Squeeze your abs for a second and then roll the ball back to the starting position. Repeat for the desired number of repetitions.

Comments: Keep the movement smooth and maintain a neutral position in the spine. In other words, don't let your hips drop. Beginners might want to practice holding a static bridge with feet on the ball before rolling the ball toward the torso.

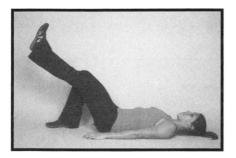

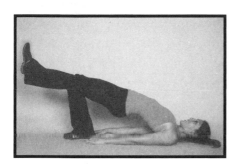

4. SINGLE-LEG GLUTE BRIDGE

This is a hip and hamstring strengthener. It teaches you to use your hips and hamstrings together, rather than your lower back, to extend your hips.

Action: Lie on your back with your arms at your sides. Bend your left knee to 90 degrees with your left foot flat on the floor. Then, while keeping your right leg straight, raise your hips so that you create a straight line from your knee through your hip to your shoulder. Maintain this position by pushing your left foot into the ground while squeezing your glutes. Hold for 30 seconds, then repeat on the other side.

Comments: Brace your midsection (abdominals) while squeezing your glutes. Beginners might want to start with both feet on the floor and gradually progress to the one-leg bridge.

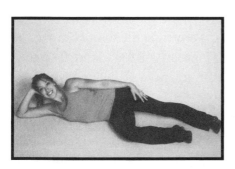

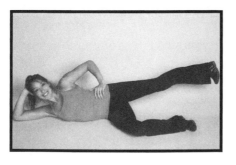

5. LYING HIP ABDUCTION

This works the gluteus medius, which stabilizes the hip during single-leg movements such as walking, running, and one-leg squats.

Action: Lie on your side with your bottom leg bent in front of you and top leg straight, with your hip slightly hyperextended. Slowly raise your thigh up and down for the desired number of repetitions. Then repeat on the other side.

Comments: Keep your hip stationary. You can check for any unwanted movement by putting your hand on your hip. You also want to keep your femur (thigh bone) internally rotated, which you can check by watching to see that the side of your foot is flat when you raise your leg.

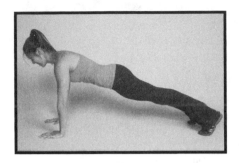

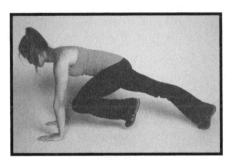

6. MOUNTAIN CLIMBERS

This is a full-body exercise that challenges both the legs and the core.

Action: Begin in a push-up position with arms straight and the balls of your feet on the floor. Brace your midsection and keep your body still. Bring your right knee toward your chest and then back down to the starting position. Repeat with your left knee and continue alternating your feet as fast as you can.

Comments: Focus on bracing your core and keeping your body balanced while maintaining a neutral spine.

PRIMAL BODY FOUNDATION EXERCISES

Now you are ready to bring the seven Primal movements, the foundation of the Primal Body functional strength program, into your exercise workout. As previously noted, the seven movements used by early humans in all their activities are the squat, lunge, bend, push, pull, twist, and gait. All functional exercises target these seven basic movements, or combinations thereof, and are built on their foundation.

The following fourteen functional exercises can be incorporated into your training routine. Use the principle of progressive overload to gradually increase your results in strength and muscle building. In Chapter 10, I will refer to these exercises in helping you design a specific regimen to fit your needs, level, and goals.

Primal Movement Exercises
EQUIPMENT: KETTLEBELL, STEP, MEDICINE BALL, PULL-UP BAR, BENCH, STABILITY BALL

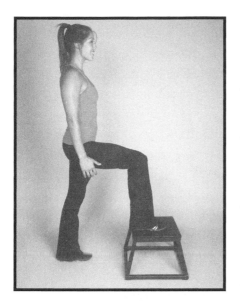

1. STEP-UPS (SQUAT)

This works every muscle in the leg. This exercise develops leg strength for running and jumping because the independent leg action of stepping up closely resembles the movement patterns of those activities. Use your body weight first and progress by using a dumbbell, barbell, or weighted vest.

Action: Place the foot of your first leg on a step. Stand on the bench by extending the hip and knee of your first leg, while your second leg rests behind your first leg without touching the bench. Lower your second leg back down to the floor. Return to the original standing position by placing your first leg on the floor. Repeat this sequence with your opposite leg, then alternate between legs for the desired number of repetitions.

Comments: Look straight ahead and keep your torso upright. Stepping closer to the bench emphasizes the quadriceps; stepping farther away from the bench emphasizes the buttocks.

STEP 4

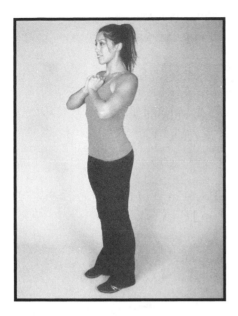

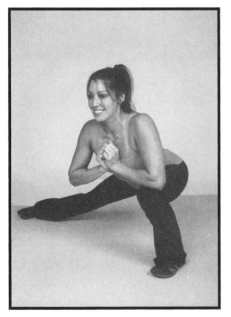

2. LATERAL LUNGE (LUNGE)

This is a frontal-plane (side-to-side) hip mobility exercise that can be used to increase range of motion when done at body weight. To improve strength, use a kettlebell, dumbbells, or a medicine ball. (This is example of progression in training.)

Action: Stand with feet together and hands clasped above your chest. Keeping your abs tight and chest high, take a big step to the left and squat down by lowering your hips down and back. Your trailing leg should be relaxed with the knee extended.

Then push off with your left leg and return to the starting position. Repeat for the desired number of repetitions on the left side and then switch to the right side or alternate back and forth between sides within the same set.

Comments: Keep your torso upright with back as straight as possible and knees behind your toes. Your shoulders, hips, knees, and feet should point forward at all times.

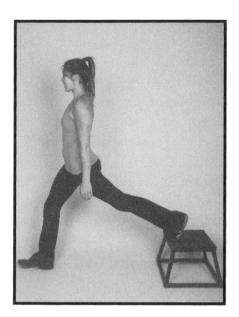

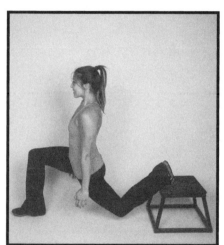

3. SPLIT SQUAT (SQUAT)

This is for improving single-leg strength and works almost every muscle in the lower body. As with most body-weight exercises, begin with no external weight, and as you advance, add dumbbells, a bar, or weighted vest to increase the difficulty (again as a progression).

Action: Position yourself with one leg out in front and the back leg raised on a step. Slowly lower yourself down by dropping your back knee down. Your front knee should bend to 90 degrees, with the shin vertical and your back knee coming close to touching the ground. Then push yourself back up to the start position. Continue for the desired number of repetitions and then repeat on the other side.

Comments: Maintain an upright posture so that your upper body is not leaning forward. Keep your chest high and shoulder blades seated down and back. Your hips, shoulders, knees, and feet should all be pointed straight ahead. Beginners may want to start with the back foot on the floor to decrease difficulty.

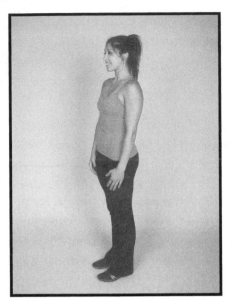

4. ONE-LEG STIFF-LEG DEADLIFT (BEND)

This develops the glutes and hamstrings while also enhancing balance and mobility.

Action: With shoulder blades down and chest elevated, raise your foot and continue to push your leg back, with knee fully extended, until your leg is parallel to the floor. Then return to the starting position and repeat for the desired number of repetitions. Switch sides and repeat.

Comments: Strive to keep your hips level throughout the entire range of motion.

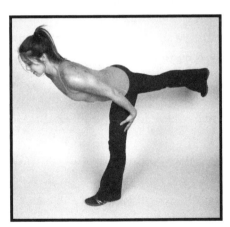

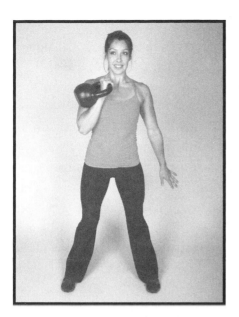

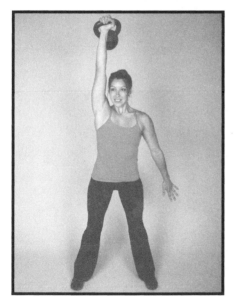

5. KETTLEBELL MILITARY PRESS (PUSH)

This is a great exercise for strengthening the shoulders, pecs, and triceps. It is also very effective at teaching you to lift as one unit (all of your joints are linked)—the essence of functional training. (For more on kettlebell training, see page 111.)

Action: Stand with your feet shoulder width apart and the kettlebell in the racked position (elbow in, hand by your shoulder, and the kettlebell resting on top of your forearm).

Tighten your glutes, abdominals, and quads, and while keeping your shoulders down, push your elbow out and up, keeping your forearm vertical, so that your hand is facing away from you and your elbow is locked out and close to your ear at the top. Lower the kettlebell down actively, by pulling it down with your lats. Pause for one second in the rack without relaxing and press again.

Comments: Avoid bending back while pressing. Keep the shoulder down and think of pushing yourself away from the kettlebell while keeping your whole body tight.

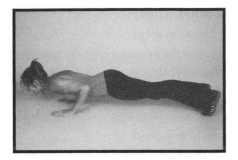

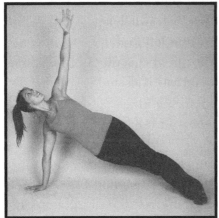

6. T PUSH-UP (PUSH + TWIST)

This is a transverse-plane (rotational) upper-body exercise that combines upper-body strength training with trunk development.

Action: Perform a traditional push-up. In the up position, balance on your right hand and rotate your body, using your core muscles, 90 degrees until your left arm is perpendicular to the floor (your body will form a T). Rotate back until the right arm is down and you are in the up position of the push-up. Then perform a traditional push-up and, upon return to the up position, repeat the process, but balance on your left hand and rotate your right arm and torso. Continue this sequence for the desired number of repetitions.

Comments: This particular push-up not only builds upper body and torso strength, it also develops shoulder stability while working in two planes of motion: the sagittal (front-to-back) and transverse (rotational) planes. Beginners may want to place their hands on a bench to decrease difficulty.

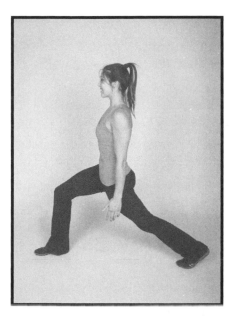

7. LUNGE JUMPS (LUNGE)

This is a plyometric exercise (involves rapid stretching and contracting of the muscle to produce power) that develops lower-body speed, strength, and leaping ability.

Action: Start in a lunge position with your right foot in front. Explode up, using both legs, and lift your body as high into the air as you can. Then switch legs in midair and land with your left foot in front and right foot behind, balancing on your toes. Continue to alternate back and forth.

Comments: This is a great exercise to use for metabolic resistance circuits, a series of multijoint movements performed in a circuit with brief, incomplete rests between exercises.

STEP 4

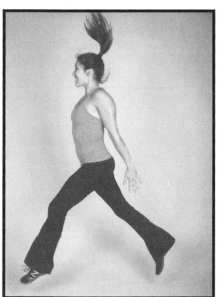

127

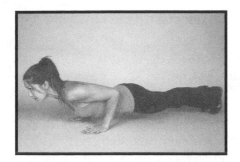

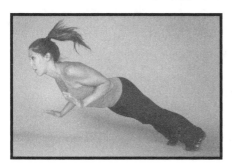

8. PLYOMETRIC PUSH-UP (PUSH)

This is a high-intensity exercise that develops upper-body strength and power.

Action: Begin in a push-up position with your arms straight and the balls of your feet on the floor. Brace your midsection, lower yourself down to the floor, and with explosive force push yourself up so hard that your hands come off the floor. Repeat for the desired number of repetitions or amount of time, if performing timed sets.

Comments: Perform this exercise on a padded surface.

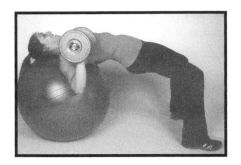

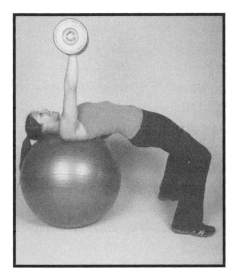

9. SINGLE-ARM STABILITY BALL CHEST PRESS (PUSH)

This strengthens the chest, abs, lower back, glutes, and hamstrings.

Action: Lie on a stability ball with dumbbell in hand, arm fully extended, opposite hand on your hip, hips level with your shoulders, knees bent, and feet flat on the floor. Lower the dumbbell with control to your chest and then press it back up while keeping your glutes tight and shoulder blades down and back.

Comments: Be sure to use a ball that is antiburst, which means that the ball will deflate slowly if it is punctured while you are on it; it will not suddenly collapse under you.

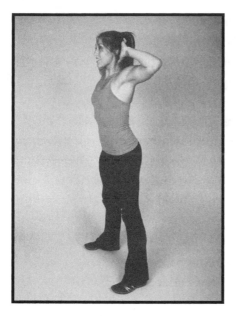

10. PRISON BODYWEIGHT SQUATS (SQUAT)

These are a slight variation on the squat Primal movement pattern.

Action: Stand with your feet slightly wider than shoulder width apart and your toes pointing slightly outward. With your hands behind your head, bend your knees and hips, keeping your back straight and knees pointed in the same direction as your feet, and descend by pushing your hips down and back until your thighs are parallel to the floor. Return by extending your knees and hips until the legs are straight and you are standing.

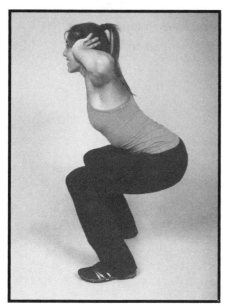

Comments: Keep your chest high and shoulder blades down throughout the movement. Maintain a natural arch in your back, brace your midsection, and don't lean forward.

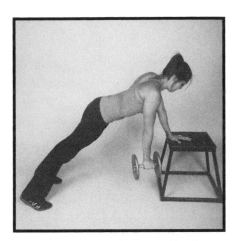

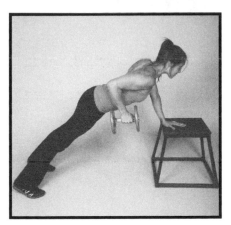

11. PRONE ROW (PULL)

This is hybrid version of the classic dumb-bell row. It works the muscles in the upper back while also developing core strength.

Action: Position yourself with one hand on a step while the other hand holds a dumb-bell, arm fully extended, with your body fully extended and your feet on the floor. Pull the dumbbell up, with elbow in, until your upper arm is just beyond the height of your back. Return to the starting position by extending your arm, and repeat for the desired number of repetitions. Then switch sides and repeat.

Comments: To maintain good form in this exercise, you need to tuck your butt. In other words, rotate the front of your pelvis toward the step, into a posterior pelvic tilt.

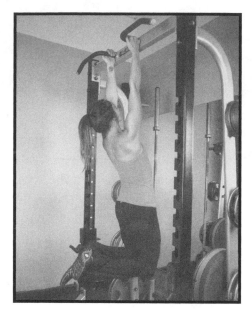

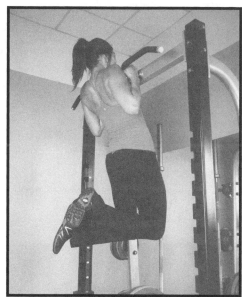

12. PULL-UP (PULL)

This is one of the best upper-body exercises for strengthening the back. The traditional pull-up uses an overhand grip (palms facing away); the chin-up uses an underhand grip (palms facing you); and in the semisupinated grip, the palms face each other. The pull-up bar should be at a height that requires you to jump up to grab it and your feet should hang free.

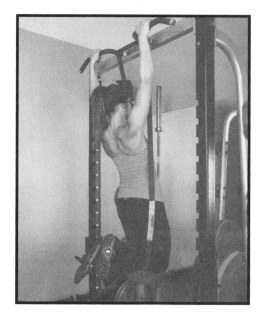

Action: Stand below the bar with your feet shoulder width apart. Jump up and grab the bar with a semisupinated grip. Pull yourself up until your chin is level with the bar. Lower yourself down until your elbows are straight. Repeat the movement without touching the floor. If you can't do one pull-up, loop a resistance band around the handles on the pull-up bar and one knee, to provide some assistance.

Comments: Steady any swinging and lead with your chest high and your shoulders down.

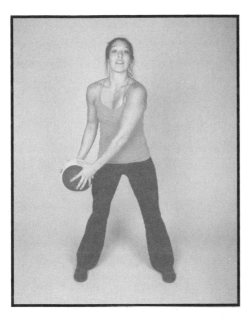

13. REVERSE MEDICINE BALL WOOD CHOP (TWIST)

This involves rotating a medicine ball across your body in a smooth, wood-chopping motion, starting with the ball on the side of your hip and ending with the ball above your head. This exercise strengthens not only your core but also your arms, shoulders, and lats.

Action: Pick up a medicine ball and move the ball up and across your body in a smooth, reverse wood-chopping motion. Your upper body should stay upright with your elbows extended, so that you are moving the weight with your torso.

Comments: Don't use more weight than you can handle.

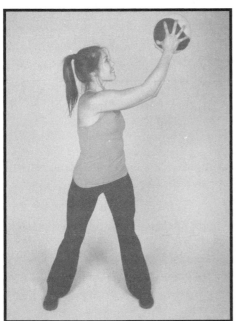

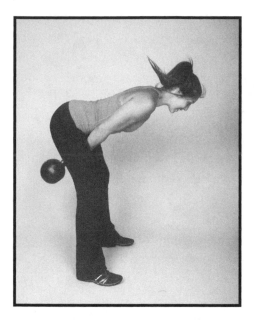

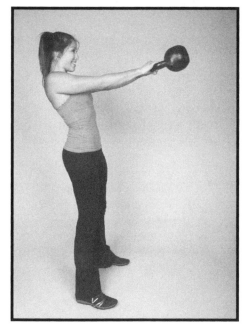

14. KETTLEBELL SWING (BEND)

This involves swinging a kettlebell back and forth between your legs and out in front of you to chest height for repetitions. This exercise teaches you to immobilize the spine while mobilizing the hips in what is known as a hinge. (For more information on kettlebells, see the box on page 111.)

Action: Stand a foot behind the kettlebell in a wider-than-shoulder-width stance, toes pointed out about 20 degrees. Sit back into your heels, grab the kettlebell with both hands, and pull your shoulders down. Start by pulling the kettlebell through your legs close to your groin and thrust the bell forward to chest height, using your hips. Squeeze your quads and glutes at the top of the movement and repeat for a desired number of repetitions or timed sets.

Comments: This is a ballistic movement and is meant to be done explosively. Be sure to keep your shoulders down and chest high to avoid rounding your back.

Rick's Transformation
Finding the Fountain of Youth

RICK is a forty-one-year old air force veteran and has been a police officer for the past eighteen years. In his own words, he tells how training the Primal way got him his stunning results.

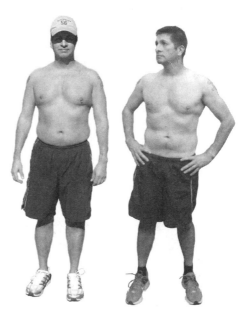

As a police officer, I've always stayed at the top of my game in physical fitness and mental stability. In my twenties and early thirties, I carried 190 pounds on my 5'8" frame. But in my later thirties, I started to slow down. I'd hit my own pinnacle of self-knowledge, working with traditional body-building techniques, and was no longer motivated to continue.

This was a problem because I was training newer officers who were half my age. I watched them do things I couldn't do anymore—but could've done ten years ago—and it made me think I was on the downside of my career. Police officers usually retire around fifty, but maybe, I thought, it was time for me to bow out gracefully.

Instead, I decided to get a personal trainer—and chose Mikki. I felt more comfortable training with a female than I did with a male, because my whole career has been male-oriented and very competitive. Mikki was no nonsense, strong, and that's what I wanted, because I like to push as far as I can. I was not disappointed. After our first meeting, I couldn't drive my car the next day, because my arms hurt so bad!

After following her program for two years, sometimes three times a week, I've gone from 190 to 155, losing 35 pounds. Now, when I interact with people as a police officer, they look at me with new respect, because I'm leaner and younger looking. When I go out on a call and people want to talk with the senior officer, they're surprised to see me, compared to another officer who's younger but a bit overweight and looking older. I look younger

than when I was thirty, and people guess I'm in my late twenties or early thirties. It makes me feel good and I want to keep going.

When I'm on duty, I carry a 25-pound gun belt, often the source of an aching back by the end of the day. Sometimes I have to chase people with all that equipment on, something I can now do without getting slowed down and winded. I'm able to end altercations more quickly and dole out punishment more effectively. But the mental and emotional aspects of my job, dealing with people's problems all day, is even more of a challenge, and being fit from both diet and exercise, I'm much more able to deal with that stress.

The dietary change on the program was hard for me at first, mainly due to my shift hours and work demands. I've noticed the leaner I've gotten and the more I work out, the less hungry I am, but still, I had to learn to plan to bring food with me and plan my meals. For example, I usually carry a couple of protein shakes, water, nuts, and pieces of protein, like meat, that I can eat cold because I'm on the go a lot. I'll also try to take a small salad and some fruit. I watch the other officers eat at

Taco Bell or McDonald's, but I haven't done that in over a year. I also no longer eat what was my favorite comfort food, bread, and a side benefit of that is I no longer have allergy symptoms from being gluten intolerant.

To say I went through a full lifestyle change, not only in working out and dietary change, but in self-confidence and self-esteem, is an understatement—I feel like a totally different person now than I did two years ago.

Kettlebell training has been a large part of my increased confidence on the job. It's helped me to strengthen my upper body to the point of making me faster, able to move laterally and front to back. In my profession, I often have to move on the spur of the moment, and KB training is great for learning fast reactions. It's also made me more limber, more agile, very flexible, and helped with endurance. I can carry my heavy equipment around for twelve hours and not feel worn out by the end of my shift.

Now, at forty-one, it's great to feel that I haven't hit my peak yet—I've got a lot more to go! It's like finding a fountain of youth—I'm aging backward as the years go by!

NEXT . . .

In the next chapter, I will show you how to do metabolic exercises to burn fat and how to combine high-intensity interval training with functional strength training for an exciting new hybrid that guarantees you will turn your body into an efficient fat-burning machine. This is the way our ancestors moved, and the way that you will find is the most natural and effective way to exercise for the best results.

Chapter 8

Step Five—Kick Up Your Metabolism to Burn Fat Faster

Whereas Step 4 emphasized the full-body movements of functional strength training, Step 5 focuses on metabolic training, also referred to as cardiovascular training. Metabolic training uses high-intensity interval training (HIIT) combined with low-intensity "play" activities, such as swimming, hiking, and walking. As you will see, it is the perfect fat-burning exercise for your genetics, mimicking the kinds of movements done by our early human ancestors.

Again, keep in mind that while you are getting an overview of the different approaches to metabolic training in this chapter, Chapter 10 will show you how to lay it all out in a plan that is customized for your individual use.

AEROBICS VS. HIGH-INTENSITY TRAINING

Step into any gym at peak times and what do you see? Treadmills, elliptical trainers, and stationary bikes all maxed out, sometimes with a waiting line. The activity most exercisers are engaged in on these machines is continuous and low intensity, commonly known as aerobics.

Very possibly, you are one of these people yourself, working out on machines regularly or maybe running a couple of times a week. Your purpose is to burn fat and stay fit. And there is every reason for you to think you are doing the right thing.

Our national devotion to cardiovascular exercise, as introduced in 1968 by Dr. Kenneth Cooper—a former air force colonel and author of the best-selling, trend-starting book *Aerobics*—has become a worldwide tradition. The Jane Fonda craze hit only a few years after Cooper, capturing millions of baby-boomer women who wanted their body to reflect fitness and health, not just shapely curves.

Ever since then, aerobic-style weight-loss and fitness exercise has been accepted without question by the general public. People today can't seem to get enough running, cycling, and dance classes, along with other extensions of traditional "cardiovascular" aerobic exercise.

But continuous, aerobic training of this kind has had its price, not only in increasing the number of knee replacement surgeries required by aging baby boomers, but in the sheer amount of time needed to accomplish any kind of results. Still, the trend persists, and in asking myself why, I can only answer that it is because of the common misconception that aerobic training is the best exercise for fat loss. In this chapter, I will show you how nothing could be further from the truth.

Traditional aerobic exercise as the mainstay of a fitness program is not congruent with how your genes were designed to be expressed, and therefore not the best for your health. Nor is low-intensity, continuous aerobic training the most efficient form of exercise for burning fat. Yes, running does burn fat, and our ancestors did run, but that kind of continuous aerobic activity was not their only— or even their primary—form of movement. Something else got them to be in a physical condition analogous to that of Olympic athletes of today.

Research clearly shows that for millions of years our Paleolithic ancestors performed movement of varying intensities, not just the long-distance, low-intensity type of traditional exercise so prevalent today. Actually, the movement patterns of early humans were predominantly high intensity, involving bursts of explosive movement rather than movement over long distances. These patterns evolved over eons of time to take advantage of specific kinds of muscle fibers and metabolic pathways most efficient at providing energy for survival, and so are a part of what we know today as the human genome.

Our ancestors performed activities of varying intensities, but their ability to perform high-intensity movements kept them in the evolutionary race. A caveman's fate could be decided in an instant by his ability to sprint from a predator or fight his way to safety. Cavewomen who could leap up onto a ledge to avoid flash floods or lava flows from volcanic eruptions lived longer. How we modern humans can mimic the activity patterns of ancestral humans is through performing high-intensity interval training.

What does HIIT look like in terms of modern human activity? While we're not likely to have predators and frequent natural disasters at our heels, we can imitate ancestral patterns by sprinting up hill in intense thirty-second bursts of movement, followed by ninety seconds of rest. And then do it again for a number of times. Another way to do HIIT is to climb a set of stadium steps at a rapid pace, followed by a period of recovery, and then repeating the climb again, interval style.

There are many other ways to do HIIT, including a hybrid form of strength training and another that gives you the best bang for your buck in time spent and calories burned, as well as protecting your joints so you can take exercise with you into your later years. There are directions for these in this chapter.

The HIIT routines I show you in this step is actually a different kind of cardiovascular training than the traditional aerobic training people have been doing since the '60s. Traditionally, people have mistakenly used the term *cardio* to describe low-intensity, aerobic exercise, such as long-distance running or cycling. *Mistakenly*, because researchers have found that the most effective cardiovascular training doesn't have to be aerobic or low intensity—it can also be high-intensity activity that is done noncontinuously, in intervals. I prefer the term *metabolic training* rather than *cardio*, because metabolic training includes both low-intensity, continuous *aerobic* training, as well as high-intensity, *anaerobic* interval training.

METABOLIC TRAINING

A new buzz word used increasingly by popular fitness gurus is *metabolism*, pointing to a very basic but rarely understood physiologic process as the key to weight loss and conditioning. But how exactly does your metabolism play a part in helping you achieve your goals? The answer lies in what I am referring to as *metabolic training*, an approach to working out in which exercises are performed to improve the efficiency of your metabolism by accessing key energy pathways.

Metabolism is defined as the set of chemical reactions that happen in living organisms to maintain life. These reactions happen through specifically organized metabolic energy pathways in which the food you eat, aided by enzymes, is transformed into energy in a series of steps. When you do metabolic training, you target each of the body's three key metabolic energy pathways through specific kinds of exercises I will show you in this chapter, maximizing your metabolism to accomplish your goals.

Here is how it works: For movement to occur, your muscles must contract, which requires energy. The energy is supplied by the food you eat—carbohydrates, fat, and proteins—when it is converted into adenosine triphosphate (ATP). Think of ATP as a usable form of energy released during the metabolic process and made available to your muscle cells for movement. Depending on the intensity of your exercise, you can access the best energy pathway to most efficiently burn fat and improve your conditioning, although the three energy pathways do not work independently of one another.

Each of the three pathways utilizes a different process to create energy, and by understanding the characteristics of the three pathways, you can better plan the appropriate work and rest intervals for the specific exercises I will show you in the second part of this chapter. The three key energy pathways are: the ATP-CP pathway, the glycolytic pathway, and the oxidative pathway:

The **ATP-CP pathway** is the most immediate source of ATP for muscular contraction. It supplies energy in the absence of oxygen (anaerobic), providing your muscles with about ten seconds' worth of energy. This pathway first uses up the ATP already stored in the muscle (two to three seconds' worth) and then it uses creatine phosphate (CP) to resynthesize ATP.

When you train using the ATP-CP pathway, you do activities of very high intensity and short duration, such as high-intensity intervals lasting six to ten seconds. Sprints are one way that your body uses this energy pathway to produce ATP. Tabata, a protocol which I will introduce later in the chapter, is another. The best way to allow the muscles to effectively replenish the CP and ATP stores is to rest during the recovery period.

The **glycolytic pathway** supplies energy through the partial breakdown of glucose, and like the ATP-CP pathway, does this without the use of oxygen, or anaerobically. This pathway provides a greater amount of energy for short, intense bursts of activity (HIIT) that can last for up to a couple of minutes. However, large amounts of lactic acid are produced as a by-product of the glycolytic pathway, until a point known as the lactate threshold is reached when muscle burn and fatigue make it difficult to continue. Training using this energy pathway involves becoming accustomed to the discomfort and fatigue that result from high levels of lactic acid in the muscles and blood. If you want to remove some but not all of the lactic acid accumulated during the work intervals, perform light activity during the rest phase of the interval, which should help with any discomfort.

The **oxydative pathway** is different than the other two pathways in that it uses oxygen (aerobic) to make ATP, the usable source of energy for the body. This pathway is slow to produce ATP, taking about two minutes, because it requires the circulatory system to transport oxygen to the working muscles before ATP can be produced. This pathway is used primarily during aerobic exercise, which is less intense and can continue for long periods of time, sometimes hours. Think running, biking, hiking, skating, and other traditional aerobic, low-intensity activities. They all access the oxidative pathway.

As I have said, the energy (ATP) produced through the three energy pathways is utilized by your muscles to create movement, and that movement depends on the type of muscle fiber making up your muscle. Two types of muscle fibers are called into action: slow twitch (ST, or type I) and fast twitch (FT, or type II). We all have a genetically predetermined mix of both types, but on average, each person has about 50 percent slow twitch and 50 percent fast twitch in the muscles we use for movement. **Fast-twitch muscle fibers** are recruited to generate short bursts of strength or speed, but they fatigue more quickly than slow-twitch fibers do. A good example of generating force rapidly is a sprint. **Slow-twitch muscles** are better suited for activities that require extended muscle contractions, as they fire more slowly and can go on for a long time before they fatigue. Slow-twitch muscle fibers are great for helping athletes run marathons or ride bicycles for hours at a time.

Now let's relate the two kinds of muscle fibers to the three pathways of energy production to get the full picture of how to use metabolic training to improve movement efficiency for your specific purpose.

For simplicity, let's group the two anaerobic energy pathways (ATP-CP and glycolytic) together, as both are utilized in high-intensity intervals (HIIT). The other pathway, the oxidative, is utilized by a slower pace of movement. The box below summarizes these differences.

The human body, as I've said, is composed of about half ST fibers and half FT fibers, the composition varying by specific muscles. Why then, if distribution of ST and FT fibers is roughly equal, do most exercise programs—recall the gym lineup for "cardio" machines—focus mainly on the ST fibers through aerobic exercise?

Clearly, this isn't the way to go. Fast-twitch muscle activation is the key to longevity and youthful movement. Research has proven that as we age and fail to use our FT muscle fibers, we lose them, limiting our ability in athletic endeavors and in basic everyday activities. The reflexes needed to catch ourselves from falling, to lift a heavy object quickly, or sprint our way to safety are no longer reliable without healthy FT muscle fibers.

Energy, Muscles, and Movement

ANAEROBIC/HIIT: When the training is characterized by short bursts of intense activity and your body uses FAST-TWITCH MUSCLE FIBERS to facilitate explosive movements.

AEROBIC: When the body uses SLOW-TWITCH MUSCLE FIBERS and produces energy at a slower pace but can sustain the production over a longer period of time.

Art De Vany's model of fitness, similar to mine, combines activities of varying intensity to mimic ancestral humans. He says the key is to hit the right balance of intensity and variety, and advises that we live in the fast-twitch muscle fiber zone, where our metabolic rate is many times our basal metabolism for intermittent, brief intervals—in other words, *train using HIIT*. Most of us today are too sedentary in our everyday routines and typically perform low-intensity aerobic exercise, never achieving the kind of metabolic peaks that were commonplace for our ancestors.

GAINING WEIGHT WITH AEROBICS

A client I trained a few years back contacted me recently to say she'd been gaining weight and needed to do something about it. When I asked her what kinds of activities she'd been doing, she told me she was inline skating along the beach in Santa Barbara every day, and that was it.

How could she be gaining weight, she asked, when the continuous, aerobic exercise she'd been doing every day was supposed to burn calories? My answer to her question came right out of Primal fitness theory and shows why aerobic activity is inferior to HIIT when weight loss is the goal.

De Vany believes that too much aerobic exercise can decrease the human growth hormone that tells your body to burn fat and build muscle. Another explanation is that high-volume aerobic training downgrades your fast-twitch muscle fibers into slow-twitch muscle fibers over time. Furthermore, aerobic training decreases your total muscle mass, which slows down your metabolic rate, so you expend less energy. Less energy expended means less calories burned, which would explain the weight gain my client was experiencing.

Obviously, it takes a while for this process to happen. With aerobic training, you'd certainly burn fat in the beginning, especially if you have been sedentary for a number of years prior to exercising. But if fat loss is your goal, a fitness program that emphasizes aerobic activity is not the best. A program that emphasizes interval and resistance training is much more effective, and it is this kind of program that forms the backbone of my Primal Body exercise program.

HIIT BURNS FAT FASTER

Scientific studies have shown how aerobic exercise compares with HIIT to bear out the importance of HIIT in the Primal Body Program. One of Australia's top fat loss researchers, Steve Boutcher, put forty-five overweight women through a fifteen-week study, where one group did intervals for twenty minutes. That group of women sprinted on a stationary bike for eight seconds, followed by twelve seconds of light cycling. The other group of women did aerobic exercise at a continuous pace for forty minutes—the more traditional approach to fat loss. Both groups exercised three times a week and had their dietary intake closely monitored. The results were that the interval group lost three times as much fat, doing half as much exercise![1]

Why did the HIIT work better to burn fat? The first group of women in Boutcher's study were doing the kind of training that causes a phenomenon called excess postexercise oxygen consumption (EPOC). As discussed on page 32, after you perform high-intensity exercise, such as sprinting on a stationary bike, your body continues to need oxygen, leaving your metabolism elevated for hours after your workout before it returns to normal. Originally referred to as "oxygen debt," EPOC is the term researchers now use to describe the events that occur as the body returns to homeostasis.

Research suggests that high-intensity training, whether you are running sprints or performing resistance circuits, disturbs the body's homeostasis, throwing the body off its normal balance. This results in a larger energy requirement after exercise to restore the body's systems back to normal. This energy expenditure causes a significant increase in fat loss, which makes HIIT the most effective method for fat loss.

Having your metabolism kick into such high gear is a key for burning fat and losing weight. In a 2002 study, European researchers found a measurable increase in EPOC thirty-eight hours after exercise. The study involved a circuit of four sets each of heavy bench press, power cleans (an explosive lift), and squats, for a total of twelve sets performed in thirty-one minutes. The researchers found that EPOC was significantly elevated up to thirty-eight hours postworkout.[2]

Thirty-eight hours is a long time for your metabolism to remain elevated after exercising. Imagine you worked out on Monday morning at 8 AM. On Tuesday evening at 10 PM, you would still be burning fat from Monday's workout! This is the reason that HIIT is so much more effective than the more traditional aerobic exercise alone, because you burn more fat *after the workout* rather than *while exercising,* the latter has always been the claim regarding aerobic exercise.

HIIT BENEFITS BEYOND FAT LOSS

HIIT has many benefits beyond fat loss that make it the ideal form of metabolic exercise for you to do at any age. These benefits include stimulating antiaging hormones (HGH), saving your muscles from being wasted as fuel, decreasing the time of working out, increasing your endurance, and protecting your joints from being worn out and injured over the years.

Antiaging effects: Interval training stimulates your body to release human growth hormone (HGH). A 2002 study in *Britain's Journal of Sports Science* showed that a thirty-second cycling sprint increased HGH levels by 530 percent. HGH is responsible for height growth in children, but once you finish growing, the hormone changes roles. HGH becomes an antiaging hormone in adults; it signals the body to burn fat and grow muscle.

Muscle protection: HIIT also protects your muscles, so you don't use them for fuel. This type of training drives your muscles to exert a lot of force, so rather than use muscle for energy, your body burns more fat and in the process spares your hard-earned muscle. This effect is evident if you compare the physique of a top sprinter to that of a top marathon runner. Sprinters physiques are well developed and highly muscular, whereas marathoners have very little muscle.

Decreased workout time: HIIT workouts don't take as much time as slower-paced, more traditional aerobic workouts do. You can complete a workout in twenty minutes or less. This can be convenient for modern-day exercisers with hectic schedules. You can get in a good workout and burn a significant amount of fat without spending a lot of time in the gym.

Increased endurance: Amazingly, HIIT is better at improving endurance than steady-state aerobics is. The Tabata protocol is the best example of how effective HIIT can be at improving aerobic capacity. Named after the Japanese researcher who developed the routine for a speed-skating team, the workout Dr. Tabata studied involves twenty seconds of maximum intensity exercise, followed by ten seconds of rest (ATP-CP is the dominant energy pathway). The cycle is repeated eight times and takes a total of four minutes.

In the Tabata study, two groups were compared: an interval group that cycled at 170 percent of its VO2 max, and an aerobic group that cycled for sixty minutes at 70 percent of its VO2 max. After six weeks, Dr. Tabata found that in the interval group the aerobic capacity had improved by 14 percent and the anaerobic capacity (which measures your speed endurance, or the duration you're able to sprint at full effort) had improved by 28 percent! The aerobic group showed an improvement in aerobic capacity of 10 percent, but there was no effect on those participants' anaerobic capacity.[3]

The Tabata protocol proved that HIIT is more effective at improving aerobic fitness than is performing aerobic work directly. And what's interesting is that these results took place on physically fit athletes.

One of the reasons this protocol is so effective is the short rest intervals between sprints. Standard interval training involves a work–rest ratio of 1 to 2 or 1 to 3. In other words, your rest interval lasts two or three times as long as the duration of the sprint. But the Tabata's work–rest ratio is 2 to 1, which means your rest periods are only half as long as the duration of your sprint. Obviously, this protocol offers a quick way to get fit in just four minutes a day. But this kind of training is very challenging, to say the least.

Joint protection: Interval training is easier on your joints than steady-state aerobic training is. One reason is that there are fewer repetitions with anaerobic exercise than with aerobic training. Also, the increased muscle mass associated with interval training translates to joint protection, which can protect you from injury.

METABOLIC RESISTANCE CIRCUITS

By now, you are probably coming on board with the kind of exercise and training that is evolutionarily compatible with your physiology, and you are ready to learn how to do it. In the remainder of this chapter, I will give you a brief orientation to a newer kind of HIIT, and then show you how best to train using this method, using metabolic resistance circuits (see page 193).

As you have seen, HIIT can be done in a variety of ways. The more traditional way is to use intervals solely for sprinting, whether on a track, on a bicycle, or in the pool. However, a new approach has emerged over the past couple of years that combines HIIT with resistance training, creating a hybrid method. In the new method, resistance training exercises, as introduced in Step 4, are performed in an interval fashion, using timed sets. This entails alternating high-intensity, all-out bursts of movement, followed by periods of rest, so you get the benefits of resistance and metabolic training in one package.

One immediate advantage of metabolic resistance circuits is the time factor. Now instead of lifting weights and then doing your metabolic workout at another time, you can get everything done in one workout by combining the two.

Another benefit is less wear and tear on your joints, when compared to traditional aerobic exercise. Typically, running a mile is about 1,500 foot strikes with forces as high as three to five times your body weight through the hip, knee, and ankle joints. That's a lot of trauma to your body. Compare that to a metabolic resistance circuit in which you perform a series of sets for the same amount of time, using a variety of upper- and lower-body exercises, where the force is less than body weight on the joints. Both exercises burn calories, but there would be less stress to your joints when using metabolic resistance circuits.

Our ancestors knew the wisdom of combining resistance training and interval training. To survive, they had to do certain intense activities that had them hit metabolic peaks, causing EPOC and giving them a natural afterburn to keep them lean and fit. For example, after hunting and catching wild game, early humans had to carry the carcass of the felled animal back to camp. This kind of activity is like performing metabolic resistance circuits: The hunters would pick up the heavy carcass, walk a short distance, then put the carcass down and rest, and then repeat this process—like lifting weights interval style—until they got back to their camp. This is a different activity than sprinting to get away from a predator or to catch wild game, but all are examples of high-intensity interval training and how our ancestors moved—movements that are coded in our genes and backed by modern science in their high degrees of efficiency.

HOW TO PERFORM METABOLIC RESISTANCE CIRCUITS

There are many ways to use the metabolic resistance circuit protocol, including the two methods I describe here, which are *timed sets* and the *Tabata protocol.*

Timed sets: With this protocol, you use timed sets of thirty to sixty seconds for each exercise. The resting interval is fifteen to thirty seconds before performing the next exercise. There are many ways to design these workouts, but to begin,

Primal Metabolic Resistance Circuit

Equipment: kettlebell, medicine ball
  Prison Bodyweight Squats (hands on head) (page 130)
  Kettlebell Swing (page 134)
  T Push-Up (page 126)
  Reverse Medicine Ball Wood Chop (page 133)
  Mountain Climbers (page 120)

THE TABATA PROTOCOL

This workout involves 20 seconds of maximum intensity exercise, followed by 10 seconds of rest. The cycle is repeated 8 times and takes a total of 4 minutes. Here are a couple of examples:

1. Lunge Jumps (page 127)
    Plyo Push-Up (page 128)
2. Kettlebell Swing (20 seconds work/10 seconds of rest) (page 134)

pick five exercises from pages 120–134 and perform the entire circuit three times with ninety seconds of rest between each round.

Here is an example of five exercises you could use. Instructions for how to design such a workout (including reps and weight loads) are in Chapter 10.

KETTLEBELL SWINGS: HEALTHIER ALTERNATIVE TO AEROBICS

If you could do only one exercise, and fat loss was your goal, the two-handed kettlebell swing is the exercise I would recommend. Simply swinging a kettlebell, using correct form, will cause you to build a great posterior chain (glutes and hamstrings) and lose dramatic amounts of body fat, while improving your cardiovascular fitness. More to the point, it's the fastest way to achieve a firm derriere (a tight butt).

And science backs me up. A study recently published in the *Journal of Strength and Conditioning* looked at the metabolic effect of swinging a kettlebell. Results showed that kettlebell swings provide a healthy alternative to traditional aerobic exercise, such as long-distance running, which can put a lot of wear and tear on the joints.

In the study, researchers at Truman State University asked ten college-aged men to swing a 16 kg (35-pound) kettlebell, using two hands, as many times as possible within a twelve-minute period. The men could rest as needed but the goal was to do as many repetitions as possible within the time frame. The researchers found that the men completed an average of 265 swings in the twelve minutes, and they worked at an average of 86 percent of their maximum heart rate and 65 percent of their VO2 max, which was measured prior to the test.

The researchers concluded that "continuous kettlebell swings can impart a metabolic challenge of sufficient intensity to increase VO2 max. Heart rate was substantially higher than VO2 during kettlebell swings. Therefore, kettlebells provide a useful tool with which coaches may improve the cardio-respiratory fitness of their athletes."[4]

If you try this workout, I suggest starting with three minutes of kettlebell swings. In a week or two, progress to six minutes of swings. Then, when you are able, perform nine minutes of swings. Continue on in this way until you can perform twelve minutes. With each and every exercise, you want to keep in mind the idea of progressive resistance. Start at a realistic level and progress gradually. (See page 134 for tips on form.)

LOW-INTENSITY AEROBICS FOR "PLAY"

In addition to pursuing high-intensity activities, our Primal ancestors performed a variety of low-intensity aerobic activities. These would have included walking for hours through meadows to gather plant foods, such as nuts and berries; walking for days to track wild game; moving camp while carrying a load to the new location; running long distances to deliver a message to a distant tribe; and swimming, dancing, and hiking for fun.

To replicate the low-intensity aerobic activities of ancestral humans, you want to include similar activities in your life, preferably done out of doors. I like inline skating along the beach in Santa Barbara, California. I also enjoy hiking in the beautiful foothills. Relaxation and enjoyment is the focus.

You may want to take a tai chi class at the park or play a game of beach volleyball or Frisbee with your friends. Maybe you prefer to go for a long walk in the hills with your dogs. Another idea would be to wear a weighted vest and go for a hike in the mountains. Or plant and tend a garden. Any of these activities would work. Just pick an outdoor activity that you like, allot some time in your schedule, and incorporate the activity into your life. It's that simple.

Our ancestors walked a lot carrying heavy weight in order to move camp and bring back as much of the kill as they could. Power walking, laden with real weight on the order of 35 to 100 pounds, is an effective modern version of what our ancestors did. Power walking with a backpack or scuba diving weights around the waist dramatically increases the intensity and effectiveness of walking. And it is about as effective as jogging for aerobic capacity, without the pounding and damage. It is what women among hunter-gatherers do when they gather.

—ART DE VANY, FROM HIS ESSAY "EVOLUTIONARY FITNESS"

Tiffany's Transformation
The Push to Recovery

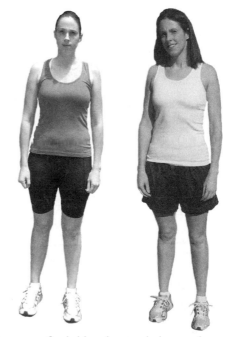

TIFFANY is a young woman who came to me after dropping out of the Police Academy training program. She'd experienced shoulder soreness that limited her ability to do push-ups, which was of concern to her trainers. An MRI showed a rotator cuff tear due to a bone spur, which she had removed surgically and then went through a five-month healing process of physical therapy and rest, before beginning to work with me.

She tells you in her own words how the Primal Body Program was part of her recovery and strengthening process that enabled her to return to the academy and eventually graduate:

I'm one of those people who believe that things happen for a purpose. When I injured my shoulder six weeks into the Police Academy, it was hard to see any light at the end of the tunnel. After surgery and a five-month recovery time, I was introduced to the Primal Body Program and Mikki through a co-worker—an event that changed my life.

One of the first things we tackled was my unhealthy eating. When we started, I ate whatever I felt like eating, which was basically a ton of carbohydrates. Pasta, bread, cookies—I was a carb lover. It was a hard transition to begin eating protein and vegetables at every meal, and very little carbs, especially sweets.

Mikki told me that after being on the Primal diet, one day I would no longer crave the sugary foods I loved so much. I remember my reply: "We shall see." I was not automatically a believer! The hardest part was breakfast, but I learned to make protein shakes in the morning. I noticed my body changed as a result of switching to the low-carb diet. My energy increased dramatically, and I felt healthier all around. Supplements also were part of my shoulder injury recovery, especially glucosamine and fish oil.

I focused on strength training with Mikki for eight months, two to three times a week, in preparation for returning to the Police Academy. I honestly never believed I'd be able to do a push-up without any pain, but I'm proud to say that I now do twenty of them, completely pain free. I also did high-intensity interval training, running up stadium steps twice a week and learning to work out with kettlebells.

Kettlebell training was a totally new experience for me. I'm not the most coordinated person on the planet, but I find swinging kettlebells a lot of fun. It sharpens my focus and challenges me to perform perfectly—I still have a long way to go. But it's entertaining, something different than what I've done for so many years, which was the more standard weight lifting.

An important part of my recovery was the foam roller. I used it to work out adhesions in my shoulder muscle from the injury, so I could do more resistance training. Now, I use the foam roller every morning to start my day, whether or not I'm training that day. It makes a big difference, because I wear a lot of weight from my vest and gun belt, and I carry it better when my muscles aren't tight.

After eight months of working with Mikki, I returned to the academy for a second try. During the class, my diet unfortunately went out the window. I had no time to shop or cook and actually gained quite a bit of weight while losing muscle mass. My hard work with Mikki had strengthened my shoulder, and then I came close to seeing it all reversed! But the experience of "falling off the wagon" was valuable in that it let me see how sticking to a Primal diet made a difference. Now, having graduated from the academy, I'm back on the Primal Program and have quickly lost the weight I gained.

Looking back over my healing and strengthening progress of the past few years, I realize that injuring my shoulder and meeting Mikki was what led me to become healthier and ultimately transform my body. I'm now so much better prepared as a police officer. My Primal lifestyle keeps me on track and in shape to do a job that I trained for and I earned!

NEXT . . .

In the next and final chapters of *Your Primal Body,* I show you how to tie together the many elements I've covered for a comprehensive plan for living the Primal Body lifestyle. You will find what you need to design a diet and exercise regime tailored to fit your fitness level. You'll also find information on how to measure your success by tracking your results. This will help you stay motivated and on track to transform your current lifestyle into one that is more in alignment with the way your body has been shaped to function over the millennia.

PART III

Putting It All Together:
Your Primal Body Plan
for Lifelong Health
and Fitness

Chapter 9

Your Primal Body Eating Plan

In Part 2, I showed you how Primal health and fitness is possible through my 5-Step Primal Body Program, each step an important module for restoring your body to genetic congruency. In Part 3, you will learn how to create a plan based on the components of my program to transform your body and live a Primal Body lifestyle for the rest of your life.

Starting with this chapter, I will show you how to design an individualized eating plan to give you the results you want, whether you are looking to lose weight or just maintain your current weight and improve your overall health. To begin your transition, I provide tools to transform your diet to a plan more congruent with your DNA; a weekly meal plan for both fat loss and maintenance on the Primal Body diet, including recipes; and a pantry list to help you shop and get started.

For most people, switching to the Primal diet takes some consideration and planning before it becomes second nature. If you have been eating the standard American diet (SAD), consisting of high carbs, bad fats, and the all-too-frequent fast-food meal, it may take a period of adjustment to get fully on board. Maybe you've been eating a vegetarian/vegan diet or a low-protein diet consisting of some low-fat animal products, whole grains, fresh fruits, dairy, and vegetables. From there, it may be a little easier to switch to a diet that is based on greater quantities of animal products, no grains or legumes, and less overall carbs.

FAT LOSS OR MAINTENANCE?

I offer two levels of the Primal Body diet, determined by your current needs. The first is for weight loss, designed to get you dropping that extra weight/fat fast. The second is a maintenance plan if weight loss is not your concern. If you want to lose weight, begin with the first level, and then once your weight loss goals are met, switch to the more moderate maintenance level.

For both levels, the starting point is to determine the amounts of each food type—protein, carbohydrate, and fat—you will be eating. The Primal Body diet is not a calorie-counting plan but a food-type plan. This is because the way your physiology has evolved, the type of food you eat is more important than the amount of calories that food contains.

Protein

Let's start with the requirements for protein. The amount of protein you need is based on your lean body mass—the portion of your body that is not fat. The basic rule is 0.8 to 1 gram of protein for each pound of lean body mass, depending on your activity level (higher levels require more protein). This recommendation takes into account the fact that the Primal Body Program includes strength training, which involves building and maintaining lean muscle mass.

It is not essential to measure your lean body mass to determine your exact protein requirements. Many of my clients start out following the guideline of eating a protein food at every meal and then being careful to avoid snacking on carbohydrates.

However, when you are first adjusting your protein intake for the Primal Body diet, a more exact measurement may be called for to predict the proper quantities of food types. The biggest challenge is to make sure you are getting enough protein, especially if you plan to go into ketosis for fat loss (revisit page 24 for more on ketosis). To maintain a state of ketosis for fat loss, you want to provide enough protein in your diet so that your body does not use your muscle to make glucose— a process called gluconeogenesis, as explained in Chapter 2.

Measuring Your Lean Body Mass

To measure your lean body mass, use a body fat caliper (see Resources, page 203) to pinch the three sites on your body, referencing the drawings on my site at http://fitnesstransform.com/assessment_of_body_composition/, and enter the data into the windows. Once you know your percentage of body fat, multiply that number by your total body weight. This number is the weight of your body fat. Subtract that number from your total weight to get your lean body mass.

Let's take for example a 100-pound woman with 25 percent body fat. Multiply her total body weight, 100 pounds, by her percentage of body fat, 0.25, to arrive at the amount of fat she has on her body: 100 x 0.25 = 25 pounds of body fat. Then subtract the 25 pounds of fat from her total weight of 100 pounds to get 75 pounds. That's her lean body mass. With a lean body mass of 75 pounds, this woman would shoot for 60 to 75 grams of protein per day to build, repair, and maintain her lean mass.

Creating a Caloric Deficit

While I stand behind the simple method of making food choices based on food types rather than the more involved method of counting calories, some people will want to know exactly how to calculate a specific caloric deficit (as mentioned in Chapter 2) for weight loss. Here is the formula I have used with my clients:

1. Create a food diary for three days, based on the foods you eat to maintain your current weight. Total the calories for the three days and divide by three to get your average daily intake.

2. Determine your protein requirements using the formula on page 154. Then multiply the number of grams by four (there are 4 calories per gram) to get the number of protein calories you require.

3. Limit your carbohydrates to 50 grams or less. Because there are 4 calories per gram of carbohydrate, your carbohydrate intake should be 200 calories or less.

4. Add the number of protein and carbohydrate calories together.

5. To determine fat intake, take the average of the three days of maintenance calories and subtract 500 calories (the caloric deficit). This is the total number of daily calories required to reach your caloric deficit.

6. Then subtract your protein and carbohydrate calories from the total number of calories needed to reach your caloric deficit. The result is the number of fat calories you require. To determine the number of grams of fat, divide by 9 (there are 9 calories per gram of fat).

Carbohydrates

The next step is to determine your level of carbohydrates. If fat loss is your goal, keeping your carbohydrate intake under 50 grams per day will get most everyone into ketosis and give you the metabolic advantage I spoke about in Chapter 2. With this approach, you can achieve a significant amount of fat loss while maintaining your lean body mass. To reach 50 grams of carbs, enjoy small portions of low-glycemic vegetables at every meal, eliminate dairy and most nuts, and skip fruits until you have reached your fat-loss goal.

If you do not have excess stored fat on your body, and maintaining a steady weight is your goal, then your carbohydrate intake will depend on your body size, activity level, and training intensity. To maintain your current weight, you may want to include some Paleo-friendly carbs, such as yams, along with low-glycemic fruits and vegetables, while still avoiding grains and sugars, such as honey, agave, and of course the ubiquitous table sugar.

Important Guidelines for Primal Meal Planning

- Eat protein at every meal. Emphasize animal protein foods from natural sources, such as organic, free-range, fresh meat, fish, and poultry, which have a healthier fat profile. Find a local supplier, if possible.

- Eliminate all grains. This includes gluten and nongluten grains, and whole and processed grains. Oatmeal is a grain. Quinoa, millet, brown rice, and corn are all grains and are not on the Primal Body diet. Grain products such as bread, cereal, pasta, pastries, and pancakes are considered grains. Go grain free!

- Include fresh, raw nuts and seeds, if you are not on a fat-loss plan. These include almonds, pecans, filberts (hazelnuts), walnuts, Brazil nuts, macadamia nuts, and pistachios, as well as pumpkin, sesame, and sunflower seeds. Raw nut butters, such as almond butter, are a good choice, too.

- Include raw, pastured dairy (if you tolerate it), such as raw cheese, yogurt, and butter, in small amounts. Avoid conventional, grain-fed dairy products. Grass-fed fermented raw milk products are an excellent source of probiotics.

- Eliminate all legumes (beans). Just like grains, legumes are a source of antinutrients, such as lectins and saponins, which wreak havoc with your hormonal and immune system. Lectins and saponins increase intestinal permeability, increasing the risk of inflammatory diseases, such as celiac disease, rheumatoid arthritis, or multiple sclerosis.

- Cut back on or completely eliminate fruit. Modern-day hybridized fruits contain high amounts of sugar, more than our Primal body can safely handle, when eaten too often and too frequently. Glycation (cellular aging) can result from too much fruit in the diet, and in general is preventable when levels of dietary sugar from all foods are lowered. When choosing fruit, choose low-glycemic fruits, as mentioned on page 56.

- Drink an abundance of water and herbal teas. Pure, filtered water is the most natural beverage available to satisfy thirst, so drink plenty of it. Men require about 3 liters per day, and women need about 2 liters. You can spice it up by adding a slice of lemon, lime, or orange to give it a citrus flavor. Or try sparkling water, which is very refreshing. Herbal teas are also a good choice on the Primal diet. Whether hot or cold, herbal teas can add variety to your beverage selection. A cup of coffee in the morning can be a great way to start the day. Coffee is brewed from the seeds of the coffee plant, not beans. And alcohol, (which was probably consumed sporadically by our ancestors) may be consumed in moderation.

Fat

The balance of your calories will come from fat. If you are on a fat-loss program, you will want to eat just enough fat to keep your energy levels up and feel sated. Once you have lost the excess fat, you will be able to consume higher quantities of healthy fat in your diet.

PRIMAL DIET TOOL: KEEP A FOOD JOURNAL

A food journal is a notebook in which you record your daily food intake. You can jot down how you feel when you are eating, to uncover any emotional triggers, or just keep it simple and write down what you ate. In either case, it's a great way to examine your eating habits.

Here are some basic guidelines:

- Carry your journal with you and write down what you eat when you eat it, rather than waiting until later and relying on memory.
- Track the date and time of day you eat.
- Note the portion size (e.g., a small bowl, fist-size, tablespoon, etc.).
- Include snacks and "just-one-bite" foods.
- Jot down any exercise you did that day.
- Update your diary every day and review it frequently. Note when you hit certain fat-loss or fitness goals, as well as when you gain weight or lose momentum, and look at the causes.

Here is a sample entry from a client's food journal

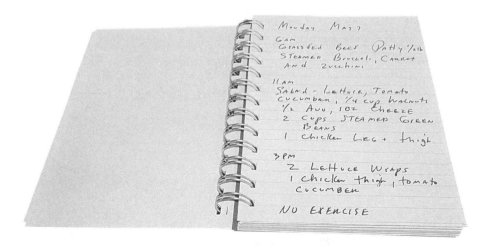

TUESDAY, JUNE 21

BREAKFAST
1 protein shake, 2 scoops protein
½ apple with 2 tablespoons of almond butter (running late)

LUNCH
2 turkey wraps with lettuce, sprouts, avocado, and honey mustard
1 small bottle of sparking water

SNACK
20 almonds

DINNER
2 chicken and steak kebabs with bell pepper
1 dinner salad with olive oil and vinaigrette dressing
1 cup of peppermint tea

WEDNESDAY, JUNE 22

BREAKFAST
1 (12-ounce) coffee with cream
3 eggs with raw cheese and spinach
2 slices of bacon

LUNCH
1 chicken breast, seasoned with rosemary
2 small raw carrots and 2 celery sticks with 2 tablespoons of ranch dressing
1 small bottle of water

SNACK
Kale chips with ½ avocado

DINNER
New York steak (8 ounces)
1 large salad with olive oil and vinaigrette dressing
2 cups of steamed broccoli
1 cup of chai tea

Healthy Snacks

INSTEAD OF . . .	ENJOY . . .
Potato chips	Kale chips (see recipe on page 183)
Crackers	Raw almonds
Pretzels	Celery sticks
Corn chips	Radishes/carrot sticks
M&M's	Macadamia nuts
Ice cream	Greek yogurt
Onion dip	Guacamole
Brownies	Berries

PRIMAL MEALS DAILY PLAN

Now that you know what to eat and what not to eat, and how to track the foods you choose with a food journal, how do you design and plan meals on the Primal Body diet? Here are a few basic ideas for breakfast, lunch, and dinner, to get you started.

Breakfast is the biggest challenge for most followers of the Primal Body diet, as it's usual to start out the day by eating grains—toast, oatmeal, or cereal. I suggest that you go to your local health food market, or possibly to Trader Joe's if there's one in your area, to find some nitrate-free, uncured bacon, and make free-range scrambled eggs to go with it. Or scramble your eggs in butter with veggies, such as onions, mushrooms, spinach, or leftover asparagus from the previous evening's dinner, and drink your coffee enriched by half-and-half or coconut milk. Fish for breakfast—a can of salmon, smoked or cured salmon fillet, or grilled fresh salmon steak—is a great way to start the day. Here's my motto: Eat dinner for breakfast and breakfast for dinner!

Lunch and dinner can follow a simple rule: a protein food plus vegetables. For lunch, have meat (beef, lamb, chicken, or fish) with a salad of raw vegetables. Alternate for dinner, by grilling your meat, fish, or chicken with an assortment of grilled vegetables. (You can use an outdoor grill, a George Foreman grill, or simply a ridged cast-iron pan coated with oil.) I like to put my meat and vegetable combination du jour into a cast-iron pot (or use my preferred "paleo pots"; see Resources, page 203), place the covered pot in the oven, and turn on the timer.

Depending on my choice, I can have a stew or roast and vegetables ready pretty quickly, or I can use a slow cooker, to have my meal ready when I come back to my house many hours later.

Preparation is simple when you are following the Primal Body diet. When I shop, I buy locally grown, in-season organic vegetables and grass-fed, hormone/antibiotic-free meats from the farmers' market. I'll also pick up some organic herbs for seasoning. Primal nutrition is easy and satisfying and doesn't require a lot of preparation. On the other hand, if you enjoy cooking, you can make foods that are flavorful by adding herbs and create your own favorite recipes. Following are one-week meal plans for both fat-loss and maintenance diets. Recipes are given on pages 168–183 for the starred (*) items.

MEAL PLANS FOR ONE WEEK

Fat-Loss Meal Plans

MONDAY

BREAKFAST
Spinach and Eggs*
Coffee or tea

LUNCH
Balsamic Chicken Breast* and Garden Salad*
Water or herbal tea

DINNER
Baked pork chop
Oyster Mushroom, Asparagus, and Onion Sauté*
Sparkling water or herbal tea

TUESDAY

BREAKFAST
Western Omelet*
Coffee or tea

LUNCH
Grilled lamb chop and Vegetable Stir-Fry*
Sparkling water or herbal tea

DINNER
Grilled Salmon* and Roasted Vegetables*
Water or herbal tea

WEDNESDAY

BREAKFAST
Grilled grass-fed beef burger with Steamed Vegetables*
Coffee or tea

LUNCH
Baked chicken breast with Sautéed Green Beans*
Sparkling water or herbal tea

DINNER
Sautéed Giant Shrimp* and Greek Salad*
Water or herbal tea

THURSDAY

BREAKFAST
Grilled sausage, sliced pear, and pecans
Coffee or tea

LUNCH
Baked ham in Garden Salad*
Water or herbal tea

DINNER
Turkey thigh with Steamed Vegetables*
Sparkling water or herbal tea

FRIDAY

BREAKFAST
Canned wild salmon on a lettuce bed
Almond butter on apple slices
Coffee or tea

LUNCH
Bacon and poached eggs
Sparkling water or herbal tea

DINNER
Grilled grass-fed rib eye steak
Steamed broccoli with butter
Water or herbal tea

SATURDAY

BREAKFAST
Grilled bison breakfast steak with scrambled eggs, mushrooms, and onions
Coffee or tea

LUNCH
Grilled Lamb Burger* with Greek Salad*
Sparkling water or herbal tea

DINNER
Salmon Roll-Ups* with celery sticks
Water or herbal tea

SUNDAY

BREAKFAST
Poached eggs
Chopped tomato, avocado, and bell pepper with olive oil and lemon juice
Coffee or tea

LUNCH
Grilled lamb chops and Sautéed Kale*
Water or herbal tea

DINNER
Roast Beef with Carrots and Pearl Onions*
Roasted Green Beans*
Sparkling water or herbal tea

Maintenance Meal Plans

MONDAY

BREAKFAST
Baked chicken breast and Sautéed Green Beans*
Pecans
Coffee or tea

LUNCH
Grilled Lamb Burger* and Greek Salad*
Water or herbal tea

DINNER
Grass–fed rib eye steak
Baked yam
Steamed broccoli with lemon–butter drizzle
Sparkling water or herbal tea

TUESDAY

BREAKFAST
Salmon Roll-Ups* with celery sticks and walnuts
Coffee or tea

LUNCH
Grilled Chicken Salad*
Sliced pear with Gruyère cheese
Water or herbal tea

DINNER
Grilled grass-fed New York steak
Grilled asparagus with lemon-butter drizzle
Red wine (1 glass) or sparkling water

WEDNESDAY

BREAKFAST
Canadian bacon with leftover asparagus, sliced tomato, and almonds
Coffee or tea

LUNCH
Grilled turkey tenders
Sweet potato
Sautéed Kale*
Water or herbal tea

DINNER
Grilled bison burger
Cold beets, Cheddar cheese, and walnuts
Sparkling water or herbal tea

THURSDAY

BREAKFAST
Veggie egg scramble with leftover sweet potato and steamed kale
Coffee or tea

LUNCH
Grilled turkey burger and Garden Salad*
Sparkling water or herbal tea

DINNER
Sautéed Cod Marinade*
Roasted Vegetables*
Macadamia nuts water or herbal tea

FRIDAY

BREAKFAST
Grilled sausage (pork, turkey, or chicken)
Cabbage Sautéed with Apples and Walnuts*
Coffee or tea

LUNCH
Grilled chicken thighs with rosemary
Baked acorn squash with butter
Sparkling water or herbal tea

DINNER
Grilled lamb chop and Roasted Green Beans*
Water or herbal tea

SATURDAY

BREAKFAST
Western Omelet* with bacon
Fruit salad (1 cup total of berries, pears, and apple)
Coffee or tea

LUNCH
Bay Shrimp Salad* with avocado
Walnuts
Water or herbal tea

DINNER
Baked pork chop
Steamed artichoke with lemon–butter dip
Sparkling water or herbal tea

SUNDAY

BREAKFAST
Spinach and Eggs* with Parmesan cheese
Coffee or tea

LUNCH
Lettuce Wrap with Ham and Cheese*
Kale Chips*
Sparkling water or herbal tea

DINNER
Grilled Salmon* on Garden Salad*
Walnuts
Mixed berries (½ cup)
Water or herbal tea

PRIMAL MEAL RECIPES

Primal Body Pantry List

SUPPLEMENTS
Whey protein powder
Super Six Supplements (see page 72)

OILS AND VINEGARS
Olive oil
Coconut oil
Balsamic vinegar
Apple cider vinegar
Red wine vinegar

SNACKS
Roasted seaweed

DRINKS
Sparkling water
Herbal teas
Coffee

CONDIMENTS
Celtic sea salt
Peppercorns
Dried and fresh herbs and spices: cumin, basil, dill, garlic, ginger, marjoram, oregano, rosemary, and thyme
Green or black, preferably organic and naturally cured olives

CANNED/BOXED GOODS
Organic free-range chicken and beef broth
Wild salmon
Sardines
Coconut milk
Tomatoes

DAIRY
Yogurt
Organic half-and-half, if you take cream
Hard, unpasteurized cheeses, such as Parmigiano-Reggiano, Gruyère, and Cheddar

NUTS AND SEEDS (PREFERABLY RAW AND UNSALTED)
Almonds and almond butter
Macadamia nuts
Walnuts
Pecans
Brazil nuts
Pistachios
Hazelnuts
Pumpkin seeds
Sunflower seeds
Sesame seeds

Egg Dishes

SPINACH AND EGGS

SERVINGS: 4

2 tablespoons butter
½ cup minced onion
1 pound fresh organic spinach, washed and chopped
8 eggs
¼ teaspoon salt

1. Heat the butter in a large skillet over medium heat and cook the onion for about 5 minutes.
2. Add the chopped spinach and cook until tender, about 5 minutes.
3. Meanwhile, in a small bowl, beat the eggs.
4. Pour the eggs into the mixture in the skillet and cook for another 5 minutes.
5. Add the salt and serve.

WESTERN OMELET

SERVINGS: 3

2 tablespoons butter
8 large eggs
¼ cup chopped and seeded green bell pepper
½ cup chopped tomato
⅓ cup chopped onion
¾ cup chopped cooked ham
¼ teaspoon salt

1. Heat the butter in a large skillet over medium heat.
2. Beat the eggs in a bowl and pour into the skillet.
3. Add the pepper, tomato, onion, and ham.
4. When the eggs have begun to set about 2 minutes, turn and cook the other side for about 2 minutes.
5. Season with the salt and serve.

Vegetable Dishes

STEAMED VEGETABLES

SERVINGS: 3

1 cup chopped cauliflower
1 cup chopped broccoli
1 cup chopped asparagus
1 cup chopped green beans
¼ teaspoon salt

1. Place about ½ inch of water in a pot with a vegetable steamer and bring to a boil over high heat.
2. Add the chopped cauliflower, broccoli, asparagus, and green beans, and cook until soft, 5 to 10 minutes.
3. Drain the vegetables, season with the salt, and serve.

VEGETABLE STIR-FRY

SERVINGS: 4

1 tablespoon coconut oil
1 cup chopped green beans
1 cup chopped zucchini
1 carrot, chopped
1 stalk celery, sliced
2 cups, ribs removed, chopped kale

1. Heat the oil in a large skillet over medium-high heat.
2. Add the green beans, zucchini, carrot, and celery, and stir-fry for about 5 minutes.
3. Add the kale, along with 2 tablespoons of water, lower the heat to medium, and cook for an additional 3 minutes.
4. Stir and serve.

ROASTED VEGETABLES

SERVINGS: 4

1 pound asparagus, chopped into small pieces
2 red bell peppers, seeded and chopped into small pieces
1 yellow summer squash, chopped into small pieces
1 zucchini, chopped into small pieces
1 red onion, chopped into small pieces
3 tablespoons extra-virgin olive oil
1 teaspoon salt

1. Preheat the oven to 450°F.
2. Toss the vegetables with the olive oil and spread in a single layer on a cookie sheet. Roast for about 30 minutes, until tender.
3. Season with salt and serve.

SAUTÉED GREEN BEANS

SERVINGS: 3

1 tablespoon butter
4 cups chopped and trimmed green beans
¼ cup sliced almonds
¼ teaspoon salt

1. Heat the butter in a large skillet over medium heat.
2. Add the green beans and sauté until tender, about 10 minutes.
3. Add the almonds, season with the salt, and serve.

SAUTÉED KALE

SERVINGS: 3

1 tablespoon coconut oil
1 clove garlic, minced
1 pound chopped kale, ribs removed
¼ teaspoon salt

1. Heat the oil in a large pan over medium heat.
2. Add the minced garlic and cook for about 1 minute.
3. Add the kale and cook until bright green, about 1 minute.
4. Add ⅓ cup of water, lower the heat, and cook for about 15 minutes, until the greens are tender.
5. Add the salt and serve.

ROASTED GREEN BEANS

SERVINGS: 3

1 tablespoon olive oil
1 pound chopped and trimmed green beans
¼ teaspoon salt

1. Preheat the oven to 450°F.
2. Spread the green beans on a cookie sheet. Drizzle with the olive oil and toss to coat evenly. Roast for 10 to 15 minutes, until crisp-tender.
3. Add the salt and serve.

OYSTER MUSHROOM, ASPARAGUS, AND ONION SAUTÉ

SERVINGS: 2

1 tablespoon coconut oil
1 onion, chopped
1 to 2 cloves garlic, minced
1 pound asparagus, chopped and trimmed
2 cups chopped oyster mushrooms
¼ teaspoon salt

1. Heat the oil in a large skillet.
2. Add the chopped onion and sauté until transparent.
3. Add the garlic, asparagus, and mushrooms. Lower the heat and cook, covered, until tender, about 10 minutes.
4. Season with the salt and serve.

CABBAGE SAUTÉED WITH APPLES AND WALNUTS

SERVINGS: 2

1 tablespoon coconut oil
2 cups chopped cabbage (use a mixture of red and green)
1 tart apple, cored and chopped
½ cup walnut pieces

1. Heat the oil in a large skillet.
2. Add the cabbage and cook for 1 to 2 minutes.
3. Add the chopped apple and cook until tender.
4. Sprinkle with the walnut pieces and serve.

Fish, Chicken, and Meat Dishes

GRILLED SALMON

SERVINGS: 1

½ pound salmon fillets
1 tablespoon melted coconut oil
Salt and freshly ground black pepper

1. Preheat a grill to medium-high.
2. Coat the fillets with the coconut oil and sprinkle with salt and pepper.
3. Cook the fish until opaque, 3 to 5 minutes on each side.
4. Remove from the grill and serve.

SAUTÉED COD MARINADE

SERVINGS: 2

MARINADE:
¼ cup olive oil
1 tablespoon minced garlic (3 to 4 cloves)
1 tablespoon minced fresh ginger
Salt and freshly ground black pepper

2 fresh or frozen (thawed) cod fillets
1 tablespoon coconut oil

1. Combine the marinade ingredients in a bowl large enough to fit the cod fillets.
2. Place the cod fillets in the bowl and marinate overnight.
3. Heat the coconut oil in a large skillet over medium heat.
4. Place the cod in the skillet. Pour the marinade over the fish, cover, and simmer for 5 to 7 minutes, until the fish is white.
5. Serve.

SALMON ROLL-UPS

SERVINGS: 1

4 ounces smoked salmon
1 ounce raw Cheddar or Gruyère cheese

1. Place the salmon fillet and cheese on a plate.
2. Roll up the fish and cheese and slice into bite-size pieces.
3. Secure each piece with a toothpick and serve.

SAUTÉED GIANT SHRIMP

SERVINGS: 2

¼ cup butter
2 cloves garlic, minced
1 pound uncooked giant shrimp, peeled and deveined
3 tablespoons freshly squeezed lemon juice

1. Place the butter and garlic in a large skillet over medium heat.
2. Add the shrimp and cook until they turn pink, about 5 minutes.
3. Remove from the heat, add the lemon juice, and serve.

BALSAMIC CHICKEN BREAST

SERVINGS: 2

2 tablespoons coconut oil
Salt and freshly ground black pepper
2 chicken breasts
2 cloves garlic, minced
¼ cup balsamic vinegar
⅓ cup chicken stock
2 tablespoons white wine

1. Heat the oil in a large skillet over medium-high heat.
2. Salt and pepper the chicken.
3. Place the chicken in the pan and cook for 3 minutes on one side.
4. Turn the chicken over, add the garlic, and cook for another 3 minutes.
5. Lower the heat; add the balsamic vinegar, chicken stock, and wine; and simmer for 10 minutes, or until the liquid is absorbed.
6. Serve.

ROAST BEEF WITH CARROTS AND PEARL ONIONS

SERVINGS: 4 TO 6

1 tablespoon coconut oil, slightly warmed

3 cloves garlic, minced

1 tablespoon Dijon mustard

1 teaspoon dried thyme

1 teaspoon dried rosemary

1 teaspoon dried marjoram

3½ pounds top sirloin beef

1¾ cups beef broth

1 cup chopped carrot (cut into bite-size chunks)

1 cup pearl onions

1. Preheat the oven to 400°F.
2. Combine the oil, garlic, mustard, and herbs in a small bowl. Coat the beef with the mixture.
3. Place the beef in a baking dish and roast at 400°F for 20 minutes.
4. Add the stock to the baking dish, lower the heat to 350°F, and roast for about 50 minutes longer.
5. Add the chopped carrot and pearl onions, and roast for an additional 20 minutes.
6. Serve.

GRILLED LAMB BURGER

SERVINGS: 3

1 teaspoon ground cumin

1 teaspoon dried thyme

Salt and freshly ground black pepper

1 pound ground lamb

1 tablespoon coconut oil

1. Add the cumin, thyme, salt, and pepper to the ground lamb.
2. Form three or four patties.
3. Coat a ribbed cast-iron pan with coconut oil. Grill the patties for 3 to 4 minutes on each side.
4. Serve.

LETTUCE WRAP WITH HAM AND CHEESE

SERVINGS: 1

2 slices ham
2 slices hard cheese
2 large romaine lettuce leaves
Mustard

1. Place one slice of ham and one slice of cheese on each lettuce leaf.
2. Add mustard to taste.
3. Roll the lettuce around the ham and cheese, secure with a toothpick, and serve.

Salads

GARDEN SALAD

SERVINGS: 4

2 to 3 cups mixed hearty greens (no iceberg lettuce)
1 celery stalk, chopped
1 red bell pepper, sliced and seeded
1 cucumber, peeled and sliced
2 tomatoes, cut into wedges
1 red onion, sliced
1 avocado, peeled, pitted, and diced
1 carrot, shredded
½ cup extra-virgin olive oil
3 tablespoons freshly squeezed lemon juice
½ teaspoon salt

1. Mix the lettuce and other vegetables in a large bowl.
2. Whisk together the olive oil, lemon juice, and salt in a small bowl.
3. Pour the dressing over the salad and serve.

BAY SHRIMP SALAD

SERVINGS: 1

1 cup fresh or frozen (thawed) tiny bay shrimp
1 cup chopped lettuce or mixed greens
1 hard-boiled egg, sliced
½ cup chopped tomato
¼ cucumber, sliced
2 tablespoons extra-virgin olive oil
2 tablespoons freshly squeezed lemon juice
½ teaspoon salt
½ teaspoon dried dill
½ teaspoon dried basil
½ teaspoon dried oregano
¼ cup grated Parmigiano-Reggiano cheese

1. Mix the shrimp, lettuce, egg, tomato, and cucumber in a large bowl.
2. Whisk together the olive oil, lemon juice, salt, and herbs in a small bowl.
3. Add the cheese, pour the dressing over the salad, and serve.

GREEK SALAD

SERVINGS: 2

1 head romaine lettuce, chopped
1 tomato, chopped
½ cup sliced red onion
1 cucumber, sliced
½ cup Parmigiano-Reggiano cheese
2 tablespoons extra-virgin olive oil
2 tablespoons freshly squeezed lemon juice
½ teaspoon salt

1. Mix the lettuce, tomato, onion, cucumber, and cheese in a large bowl.
2. Whisk together the olive oil, lemon juice, and salt in a small bowl.
3. Pour the dressing over the salad and serve.

GRILLED CHICKEN SALAD

SERVINGS: 1

1 grilled chicken breast or thigh
Garden Salad (page 180) or Greek Salad (page 181), reserving dressing

1. Slice the chicken into long, thin pieces.
2. Top your choice of salad with the chicken slices.
3. Pour the dressing over the salad and serve.

Snacks

KALE CHIPS

SERVINGS: 4

1 bunch kale, ribs removed
1 tablespoon olive oil
1 teaspoon salt

1. Preheat the oven to 350°F.
2. Chop the kale into bite-size pieces. Drizzle with the olive oil.
3. Place the kale on a cookie sheet and bake for about 15 minutes, or until crisp.
4. Sprinkle with the salt and serve.

SUPPLEMENTING FOR PRIMAL NUTRITION

You want to include the Super Six supplements I presented in Chapter 2 in rounding out your Primal Body diet, so that you can approximate the nutrient density of the diet our ancestors ate. I've listed them here, with recommended dosages, for your convenience.

If you are not used to taking quite as many supplements, here's how to get them all into your day without becoming overwhelmed and then forgetting to take them: In the morning (or the night before), divide the total pills between three containers—one container for each meal—and keep near your eating area. At each of your three meals, take the portioned amount with your food.

- Omega-3—enough to create a 2:1 ratio of omega-6 to omega-3. Spread out equally with meals.
- Vitamin D—2500 to 5,000 IU. Spread out with meals, if possible.
- Antioxidants
  ○ Vitamin E—400 to 800 IU. Take with omega-3.
  ○ Vitamin C—500 to 1,000 mg. Spread out equally with meals.
  ○ Coenzyme Q10—100 mg. Take early in day, due to energizing effect.
- Magnesium—400 to 1,000 mg. Spread out equally with meals.
- Multinutrient formula—as suggested. Take early in day due to energizing effect of B vitamins.
- Glucosamine—as needed, for painful joints. Take with or without meals.

NEXT . . .

At the same time you are implementing your new plan for Primal Body fat loss, nutrition, and supplementation, you can begin to initiate the physical activity section of the Primal Body Program for the full comprehensive approach. In this next chapter, I will show you how to design your Primal Body strength-training sessions; metabolic activities (HIIT); and "play," or low-intensity activities.

Chapter 10

Your Primal Body Fitness Plan

In my many years of consulting with clients to design their individual plans, I occasionally come across a person who tells me he or she only wants to have an exercise component and is not interested in the diet. My response is that to get all of the benefits of the program, you want to do both. Why adapt Primal movement in your workout but then ignore your DNA's requirements for fueling that workout most efficiently?

The Primal Body Program is a fundamental and comprehensive approach that will return your body to its Primal state—lean, fit, and healthy. Only then can you count on getting results that will be long lasting, because what you're doing is congruent with your genetic blueprint and therefore easy and natural to maintain.

In this chapter, I will show you how to design a Primal Body Fitness Plan for your level, and then tailor that program to fit your individual needs and goals.

For example, you may be a beginner in fitness and want to lose weight to improve your health and appearance. Or you may be starting at an intermediate level and want to build muscle so you can perform in a chosen athletic activity. As an advanced person, you may want to train more intensely but spend less time in the gym. All of these goals and more are possible with the Primal Body Program and can be met by following a regimen you design with my help to achieve your specific goals.

PRIMAL MOVEMENT AND TRAINING

Keeping in mind that we evolved to perform Primal movements, emphasizing full body exercises, the Primal Body Program is based on this model. In our modern world, we don't have the same challenges that our ancestors faced (e.g., we don't need to carry a carcass back to camp to eat), but we can look to early humans for the amount and types of exercise we evolved to perform and then replicate these activity patterns in the training environment.

When designing a program for your level and goals, where do you start? The following assessment questionnaire will help you find your entry level for the movement/training portion of the Primal Body Program, depending on how sedentary or active you have been. Once you have placed yourself in the level appropriate to your fitness and goals, you are ready to get started.

YOUR SESSION DESIGN

The first part of your Primal Body training is a strength-training workout session you perform either at home or at a club you join. This workout is designed according to a template of activities to be done at each session, beginning with a mobility drill or dynamic warm-up; followed by core strengthening, and then the mainstay of the program, Primal movement exercises; followed by foam rolling and stretching to keep the tissue healthy and flexible. (Refer to Chapters 6 and 7 for more detailed descriptions of these activities.)

For easy reference, the basic four-part template for each workout session looks like this:

1.   Mobility for warm-up
2.   Core strengthening
3.   Primal movement exercises
4.   Foam roll and stretch

In addition to your strength-training workout session, you want to include in your program a segment of metabolic training, including high-intensity interval training, as well as "play" activities. For example, an HIIT activity could consist of sprinting uphill in intense, thirty-second bursts of movement, followed by ninety seconds of rest, repeated X number of times (depending on your level). Another HIIT activity is climbing a set of stadium steps rapidly, followed by a period of recovery, and then repeating. Low-intensity play activities would include hiking, swimming, skating, and so on. (See Chapter 8 for a more detailed list of both high-intensity interval training and low-intensity play activities.)

Here is a sample of how such a workout plus HIIT/play might look for the different levels.

Tier 1: Three strength-training sessions in the gym and two lower intensity metabolic sessions (about forty-five minutes total), gradually building up to HIIT. (I almost never start my Tier 1 people out on high-intensity intervals. Most beginners are not strong enough to perform high-intensity activities but can build

Where Do I Start?

Answer the questions by assigning a value of 0 to 4. Zero is essentially "never," 1 is "rarely," 2 is "sometimes," 3 is "almost always," and 4 is "always." Add your total score and use that number to place yourself in one of three levels: Tier 1–Beginner (0–12 points); Tier 2–Intermediate (13–26 points); or Tier 3–Advanced (27–40 points).

Rate your entry level for the training program:

1. Have you transformed your physique with diet and/or exercise? 0 1 2 3 4
2. Rate your strength level. 0 1 2 3 4
3. Have you worked with a coach or trainer? 0 1 2 3 4
4. Rate your flexibility. 0 1 2 3 4
5. Do you enjoy a regular physical activity for fun: skate, bike, play Frisbee? 0 1 2 3 4
6. Rate your core strength. 0 1 2 3 4
7. Have you ever competed in sport activities? 0 1 2 3 4
8. Rate your level of coordination. 0 1 2 3 4
9. Are you free of physical problems that might limit your activity? 0 1 2 3 4
10. Rate your cardiovascular fitness. 0 1 2 3 4

My score: _____ My Tier: _____

up to it in time.) Lower-intensity activities include brisk walking up hills, hiking, or cycling.

Tier 2: Two strength-training sessions in the gym, two HIIT sessions, and one play session, such as light jogging at the beach or around the neighborhood, or playing tennis.

Tier 3: Three strength-training sessions in the gym, two HIIT sessions on alternate days of the week, and one low-intensity play activity, such as inline skating.

(You'll find charts detailing all these activities on pages 189–196.)

The foam rolling and stretching component of the template can be incorporated in a variety of ways and is useful in preparing you overall for your Primal Body training program. Regardless of your level, when you first begin this program, you will want to go through the entire series of Self-Myofascial Release modalities and all of the stretches two or three times a week, to release the chronic muscular tension and restrictions in your body (refer to Chapter 6). After you have become familiar with the SMR exercises and stretches, and you know where you store your tension, you can probably stay loose with a few SMR exercises and stretches at the end of each strength-training session, while periodically going through the entire series. But if you come into a training session feeling tight, you may want to foam roll at the beginning of the session to loosen up and then stretch after your workout, to lengthen the muscles you put under stress while exercising and improve overall recovery.

All three segments of your training are important: strength training and both types of metabolic exercise—high and low intensity. You want to design a fitness program that includes all of these on a weekly basis. For example, Tier 2 performs strength training two times weekly, HIIT twice weekly, and low-intensity play activities once a week.

Here is one way to structure that program in your weekly calendar: Perform strength training on Monday and Thursday; HIIT on Tuesday and Friday, and on Saturday, low-intensity play activities. Rest on Wednesday and Sunday. It's important to allow at least one recovery day between strength-training sessions, and always take one day a week to rest.

SAMPLE STRENGTH-TRAINING SESSIONS

The strength-training program works just as well for high-level athletes as it does for those who are beginning an exercise program. Men and women at all levels experience results because all of the exercises can be modified, based on individual fitness levels.

I'll take you through two strength-training workouts for each of the three tiers, so that you can see how they work. Refer to the exercise descriptions and photos in Chapter 7.

Strength Workout Session A

EQUIPMENT: BENCH, DUMBBELL (DB), MEDICINE BALL

TIER 1

COMPONENT	EXERCISE	SETS/REPS/TIME	REST
Mobility	Jumping Jacks	2 sets/10 reps	15 secs
Core	Lying Hip Abduction	1 set/ 20 reps	5 secs
Core	Prone Bridge	1 min hold	15 secs
Core	Mountain Climbers	2 sets/10 reps	15 secs
Primal Movement	Split Squat (back leg on floor)	2 sets/10 reps each	60 secs
Primal Movement	One-Leg Stiff-Leg Deadlift	2 sets/12 reps each	60 secs
Primal Movement	T Push-Up (hands on bench)	2 sets/6 reps each	60 secs
Primal Movement	DB Prone Row (moderate weight)	2 sets/10 reps each	60 secs
Primal Movement	Reverse Medicine Ball Wood Chop (light)	2 sets/8 reps each	60 secs
Foam Roll and Stretch	Problem/tight areas	10 mins	

TIER 2

COMPONENT	EXERCISE	SETS/REPS/TIME	REST
Mobility	Jumping Jacks	2 sets /15 reps	15 secs
Core	Lying Hip Abduction	1 set/ 25 reps	15 secs
Core	Prone Bridge (one leg)	1 min hold each	15 secs
Core	Mountain Climbers	2 sets/15 reps	15 secs
Primal Movement	DB Split Squat (back leg on bench)	2–3 sets/8 reps each	60 secs
Primal Movement	One-Leg Stiff-Leg Deadlift (DB in opposite hand of working leg)	2–3 sets/8 reps each	60 secs
Primal Movement	T Push-Up (hands on floor)	2–3 sets/6 reps each	60 secs
Primal Movement	DB Prone Row (heavy weight)	2–3 sets/10 reps each	60 secs
Primal Movement	Reverse Medicine Ball Wood Chop (moderate weight)	2–3 sets/8 reps each	60 secs
Foam Roll and Stretch	Problem/tight areas	10 mins	

	TIER 3		
COMPONENT	**EXERCISE**	**SETS/REPS/TIME**	**REST**
Mobility	Jumping Jacks	2 sets /20 reps	15 secs
Core	Lying Hip Abduction	1 set/ 35 reps	15 secs
Core	Prone Bridge (opposite arm/leg)	1 minute hold each	15 secs
Core	Mountain Climbers	2 sets/ 25 reps	15 secs
Primal Movement	Split Squat (DB on opposite shoulder of working leg)	3 sets/12 reps	60 secs
Primal Movement	One-Leg Stiff-Leg Deadlift (DB in opposite hand of working leg)	3 sets/8 reps each	60 secs
Primal Movement	T Push-Up (hands on floor)	3 sets/10 reps each	60 secs
Primal Movement	DB Prone Row (heavy weight)	3 sets/5 reps each	60 secs
Primal Movement	Reverse Medicine Ball Wood Chop (heavy)	3 sets/8 reps each	60 secs
Foam Roll and Stretch	Problem/tight areas	10 mins	

NOTES

_____

_____

_____

_____

_____

_____

_____

_____

Strength Workout Session B
EQUIPMENT: KETTLEBELLS (KB), STABILITY BALL, STEP, PULL-UP BAR, BAND

TIER 1

COMPONENT	EXERCISE	SETS/REPS/TIME	REST
Mobility	Joint Rotations	8 rotations each	15 secs
Core	Single-Leg Glute Bridge (use two legs)	1 set/12 reps	15 secs
Core	Side Bridge (bottom knee bent)	1 set/20 reps	15 secs
Core	Stability Ball Plank	30-sec hold	15 secs
Primal Movement	Step-Ups (low step)	2 sets/12 reps	60 secs
Primal Movement	KB Military Press (light)	2 sets/6 reps	60 secs
Primal Movement	Pull-Up (with band)	2 sets/5 reps	60 secs
Primal Movement	Lateral Lunge	2 sets/8 reps	60 secs
Primal Movement	KB Swing (light)	2 sets/10 reps	60 secs
Foam Roll and Stretch	Problem/tight areas	10 mins	

TIER 2

COMPONENT	EXERCISE	SETS/REPS/TIME	REST
Mobility	Joint Rotations	8 rotations each	15 secs
Core	Single-Leg Glute Bridge	1 set/12 reps	15 secs
Core	Side Bridge	60-sec hold each	15 secs
Core	Stability Ball Jackknife	1 set/15 reps	15 secs
Primal Movement	DB Step-Ups (medium step)	2–3 sets/12 reps	60 secs
Primal Movement	KB Military Press (moderate)	2–3 sets/6 reps	60 secs
Primal Movement	Pull-Up	2–3 sets/8 reps	60 secs
Primal Movement	Lateral Lunge	2–3 sets/8 reps	60 secs
Primal Movement	KB Swing	3/30-sec intervals	30 secs
Foam Roll and Stretch	Problem/tight areas	10 mins	

TIER 3			
COMPONENT	*EXERCISE*	*SETS/REPS/TIME*	*REST*
Mobility	Joint Rotations	8 rotations each	15 secs
Core	Single-Leg Glute Bridge (one leg/3 steps up)	1 set/12 reps each	15 secs
Core	Side Bridge	90-sec hold each	15 secs
Core	Stability Ball Jackknife (w/push-up)	2 sets/10 reps	15 secs
Primal Movement	DB Step-Ups (high step)	3 sets/12 reps	60 secs
Primal Movement	KB Military Press (heavy)	3 sets/8 reps	60 secs
Primal Movement	Pull-Up	3 sets/12 reps	60 secs
Primal Movement	KB Lateral Lunge (bell at chest)	3 sets/8 reps each	60 secs
Primal Movement	KB Swing	5/30-sec intervals	30 secs
Foam Roll and Stretch	Problem/tight areas	10 mins	

NOTES

_____

_____

_____

_____

_____

_____

_____

_____

HIIT/PLAY TRAINING PROGRAM

I offer two methods of HIIT: *intervals* and *metabolic resistance circuits*:

Intervals consist of sprinting uphill, for example, in intense, 30-second bursts of movement, followed by thirty to ninety seconds of rest, repeated X number of times (depending on your level). This is a basically a fifteen- to-twenty-minute workout consisting of eight to fifteen sprints, with brief rests in between. Keep in mind that the goal is *intensity*, not *duration*. You want to sprint as hard and fast as you can, not hold back or pace to "save yourself" so you can do more.

Intervals can be done in the activities of swimming, inline skating, running, power walking, cycling, or running the bleachers at your local college or high school track. You can also use your favorite cardio machine—the stair stepper, treadmill, cycle, or elliptical trainer—for interval training.

Primal metabolic resistance circuits consist of a series of exercises using timed sets of thirty to sixty seconds for each exercise, then resting for fifteen to thirty seconds before performing the next movement. Perform the entire circuit three times with ninety seconds of rest between each round. Try to do as many reps as possible within the time frame. (See Chapter 7 for a description of each exercise).

HIIT (SPRINTING UPHILL)	INTERVALS	WORK/REST
Tier 1	8	30 secs/90 secs
Tier 2	8–10	30 secs/60 secs
Tier 3	10–15	30 secs/30 secs

Metabolic Resistance Circuit A
EQUIPMENT: KETTLEBELL, MEDICINE BALL, BENCH

TIER 1	
EXERCISE	*WORK/REST**
Prison Bodyweight Squats (hands on head)	30 secs/30 secs
Kettlebell Swing	30 secs/30 secs
T Push-Up (hands in bench)	30 secs/30 secs
Reverse Medicine Ball Wood Chop	30 secs/30 secs
Mountain Climbers	30 secs/30 secs
*Rest for 90 seconds and repeat for a total of 3 rounds.	

TIER 2	
EXERCISE	*WORK/REST**
Prison Bodyweight Squats (hands on head)	45 secs/15 secs
Kettlebell Swing	45 secs/15 secs
T Push-Up	45 secs/15 secs
Reverse Medicine Ball Wood Chop	45 secs/15 secs
Mountain Climbers	45 secs/15 secs
*Rest for 90 seconds and repeat for a total of 3 rounds.	

TIER 3	
EXERCISE	*WORK/REST**
Prison Bodyweight Squats (hands on head)	60 secs/15 secs
Kettlebell Swing	60 secs/15 secs
T Push-Up	60 secs/15 secs
Reverse Medicine Ball Wood Chop	60 secs/15 secs
Mountain Climbers	60 secs/15 secs
*Rest for 90 seconds and repeat for a total of 3 rounds.	

Metabolic Resistance Circuit B

EQUIPMENT: STEP, KETTLEBELL, MEDICINE BALL, STABILITY BALL

TIER 1

EXERCISE	WORK/REST*
Split Squat (rear foot on floor)	30 secs/30 secs
Kettlebell Swing	30 secs/30 secs
Reverse Medicine Ball Wood Chop	30 secs/30 secs
Lunge Jumps	30 secs/30 secs
Stability Ball Jackknife	30 secs/30 secs
*Rest for 90 seconds and repeat for a total of 3 rounds.	

TIER 2

EXERCISE	WORK/REST*
Split Squat (rear foot on step)	45 secs/15 secs
Kettlebell Swing	45 secs/15 secs
Reverse Medicine Ball Wood Chop	45 secs/15 secs
Lunge Jumps	45 secs/15 secs
Stability Ball Jackknife	45 secs/15 secs
*Rest for 90 seconds and repeat for a total of 3 rounds.	

TIER 3

EXERCISE	WORK/REST*
Split Squat (rear foot on step)	60 secs/15 secs
Kettlebell Swing	60 secs/15 secs
Reverse Medicine Ball Wood Chop	60 secs/15 secs
Lunge Jumps	60 secs/15 secs
Stability Ball Jackknife	60 secs/15 secs
*Rest for 90 seconds and repeat for a total of 3 rounds.	

Low-intensity "play" activities include walking, hiking, easy cycling, or whatever you enjoy. The emphasis is on enjoyment! (See Chapter 8 for more suggestions.)

TIER 1 PROGRAM

WEEK	SUNDAY	MONDAY	TUESDAY	WEDNESDAY	THURSDAY	FRIDAY	SATURDAY
1	Off	Strength Workout A	Brisk walking uphill	Strength Workout B	Cycling	Strength Workout A	Off
2	Off	Strength Workout B	Inline skating	Strength Workout A	Metabolic Resistance Circuit or sprints	Strength Workout B	Off

TIER 2 PROGRAM

WEEK	SUNDAY	MONDAY	TUESDAY	WEDNESDAY	THURSDAY	FRIDAY	SATURDAY
1	Off	Strength Workout A	Metabolic Resistance Circuit A	Off	Strength Workout B	High-intensity sprints	workout Jogging
2	Off	Strength Workout A	High-intensity sprints	Off	Strength Workout B	Metabolic Resistance Circuit B	Frisbee

TIER 3 PROGRAM

WEEK	SUNDAY	MONDAY	TUESDAY	WEDNESDAY	THURSDAY	FRIDAY	SATURDAY
1	Off	Strength Workout A	Metabolic Resistance Circuit A	Strength Workout B	High-intensity sprints	Strength Workout A	Dance class
2	Off	Strength Workout B	High-intensity sprints	Strength Workout A	Metabolic Resistance Circuit B	Strength Workout B	Tennis

Chapter 11

Your Primal Body
for Life

MEASURING YOUR RESULTS

Keeping your eye on the results produced by sticking to your new program is an important way to know beyond a doubt that what you're doing is working. It will also help you stay motivated.

I recommend that you monitor your results and get involved with the outcomes you are causing. If you became the proud owner of a new Ferrari, for example, wouldn't you be meticulous about checking oils and fluids, getting the proper tune ups and tests?

Blood work is one of the most valuable tools western medicine has to offer. It can provide an accurate measurement of the changes your body goes through when you alter your nutrition and/or exercise program, the level of inflammation in your body, how well you are aging, and how well you are managing your stress. I recommend getting blood work done before embarking on the program, and then annually along the way.

Staying on top of your blood work is another way (in addition to a Primal diet and exercise) that you can begin to take an active role in your health. With today's health-care system, I believe that you have to be your own best advocate; you can't depend on your doctor.

Some of the standard tests most doctors order include total cholesterol, HDL cholesterol, LDL cholesterol, glucose, and triglycerides, which you are probably familiar with. But you'll want to request tests for LDL particle size, C-reactive protein (CRP), and glycated hemoglobin, in addition to the basics he/she recommends. (I will discuss these less familiar tests.)

In looking at the lipid panel, there are a couple of key values you'll want to pay attention to. According to Dr. Michael Eades, the lipid parameters of most importance in determining risk for heart disease are triglyceride and HDL levels. In particular, the best indicator of health is a low triglyceride-to-HDL ratio (TGL/HDL); below 2 is considered ideal.

Triglycerides are a measure of circulating blood fats. When your liver and muscles are full of glucose, the excess glucose is converted to fat in the liver and stored in the body as adipose tissue. If your triglyceride levels are high, you can be pretty sure you are eating too much carbohydrate, and you may be moving in the direction of insulin resistance and disease. So, you want to keep this value low. The reference range on the lab results suggests a level under 150 mg/dl. I have found that many who follow the Primal Body Program have values under 50 mg/dl. HDL is the good cholesterol; it carries cholesterol away from the arteries and back to the liver to be excreted away from the body in bile. You want to keep this value high, above 50 mg/dl or better.

LDL cholesterol is the bad cholesterol (think *L* for *lousy*), the kind that deposits cholesterol on the artery walls, which can lead to a narrowing of the arteries and increase the risk for heart disease. But remember, all LDL particles are not equal; the large, fluffy particles are harmless, whereas the small, dense particles do more damage. The small, hard kind of LDL cholesterol (associated with elevated triglyceride levels) is believed to be the cause of atherosclerosis, since the small, dense particles can squeeze between tiny gaps in the arterial walls and get stuck to cause harmful buildup of plaque. The large, fluffy kind of LDL cholesterol is not atherosclerotic and therefore does not predict heart disease. Because of these differences, it is important to note that particle size predicts the risk for heart disease more accurately than simply measuring your total LDL cholesterol.

In Chapter 4 on the anti-inflammatory diet, I discussed the importance of controlling inflammation in your body. Testing for C-reactive protein measures the overall level of inflammation in your body. High levels of CRP are often caused by infections and/or chronic disease.

The glycated hemoglobin test measures the amount of sugar that is sticking to your red blood cells. As this measure is related to the age of the red blood cells, it determines the average glucose level over the previous two to three months, as compared to a glucose blood test, which reflects your glucose measurement over the previous twelve hours.

One reason the glycated hemoglobin test is so valuable is that if glucose is sticking to your red blood cells, you can be sure that it is also sticking to your proteins. You may recall our discussion of advanced glycation end products (AGEs) in Chapter 4 and how, through a process of cross-linking, they cause intercellular damage, resulting in age-related disease. This test measures not only your glucose levels but also the level of AGEs in your body, which are associated with loss of vision, reduced muscular function, Alzheimer's, cardiovascular disease, and many other conditions.

Body composition measurement: One of the best ways to determine your level of fitness is to measure your body composition. The human body is composed of lean body mass—metabolically active tissue, such as bones, muscles, the brain, and organs—and fat or adipose tissue, which is nonmetabolically active tissue.

Most people use a standard scale to measure weight, but the scale does not tell you the ratio of your lean body mass to fat. Why is this ratio important? Because an athlete with 10 percent body fat may be considered overweight, according to a standard weight chart, when he is actually in excellent condition—his lean body mass–to–fat ratio is very good.

Hydrostatic (underwater) weighing, in which an individual is weighed while submerged in a large tank of water, is considered the gold standard for measuring body composition. But because this method is impractical, I prefer skinfold measurements, using a body fat caliper (which can be purchased at http//fitnesstrans form.com/store/) and entering the data into the formulas provided on my website at http://fitnesstransform.com/assessment_of_body_composition/.

What is the ideal percentage of body fat? Women tend to carry more body fat than do men, and most fitness professionals consider 14 to 18 percent to be excellent for women; and 18 to 22 percent is considered good. For men, 10 to 14 percent is considered excellent; and 14 to 18 percent is considered good. Over 22 percent for women and over 18 percent for men would be considered excessive. If you are sedentary (Tier 1), you may have 25 percent, if you are male, and 35 percent, if you are female.

Photos: Amazingly, many people who start a fitness and/or nutritional program never take "before" photos. This is a step I never miss with my new clients (as long as they agree) because photos clearly document the clients' progress.

Once you have the before photo, you might want to update that photo every month, every three months, once a year, or when you have reached your goal. I like to start with a before photo and a baseline body composition measure. Then I'll measure percentage of body fat and take a "progress" photo every three months, when I see changes, or when the client requests it. The changes in body composition and/or the visible progress from photos can be extremely motivating.

STAYING INSPIRED AND MOTIVATED

Designing and implementing a Primal Body Fitness Program is a first step toward a lifelong transformation of your body and health. Congratulations! Along the way, it's natural that you may become discouraged and occasionally relapse—you're only human! To stay on track and maintain your newly transformed body, you must find ways to keep motivated and inspired.

Find support. One of the keys to success is to surround yourself with people who are living the Primal lifestyle. I encourage you to interact with my website, http://fitnesstransform.com/, for support and motivation.

Work with a personal trainer. Scientific research supports that working with a trainer is highly beneficial. A recent study compared the effects of exercising with a trainer, to exercising without one but getting advice. In this four-month study, one group met with a trainer twice a week; the other group received advice about training and had access to a fully equipped gym but lacked supervised instruction. The researchers found that members of the group that worked with the trainer lost almost 10 pounds more fat—a total of 13.6 pounds while the unsupervised group lost only 3.7 pounds each. And this was without any changes in diet.

So if you are serious about changing your body, consider hiring a coach—someone who can help you reach your goals. I find that most people need advice. They also need someone to be accountable to. I can't tell you how many times I've heard the words "If you weren't standing there, I'd never do this."

So how do you find a good trainer? What do you look for? Obviously, a trainer must have knowledge. One of the more rigorous certifications to look for is the National Strength and Conditioning Association's (NSCA) Certified Strength and Conditioning Specialist (CSCS). This certification requires the trainer to have at least a bachelor's degree to qualify for the test, and it ensures that the trainer/coach has a basic understanding of biomechanics, exercise physiology, and program design.[1]

You also want to look for a trainer who uses foot-based, functional/Primal movements in combination with high-intensity interval training to build muscle and burn fat. This is the best way to reach your goals following the Primal Body Program, not the more traditional approach of isolating muscles on machines and low-intensity cardiovascular training emphasized in so many gyms.

One thing you want to be aware of is that the fitness industry is not standardized. Because of this, you as a consumer are vulnerable to rip-offs. Fit-looking trainers with fly-by-night certifications are ubiquitous. If you do decide you want to work with a trainer, do your research and make sure that whoever you hire is qualified to help you.

If you can't afford a personal trainer . . . If for whatever reason, working with a personal trainer on a weekly basis isn't for you, then consider hiring a coach once per month and use him or her as a consultant to design your monthly fitness program. Maybe you have a friend with some knowledge of fitness, with whom you can work out to explore the Primal Body Program laid out in this book. And then again, perhaps you want to go it on your own. The good news is that all of these approaches will lead to success if you make the commitment and follow through. Then one day, when you've reached your health and fitness goals, you'll look back to the day when you first started, hopefully marked by a photo of the former you, and realize how far you've come.

LOOKING AHEAD . . .

In the fitness world, the first six weeks of your training is known as the "drawing-in" period. Somewhere between the third and sixth week, a wonderful metamorphosis takes place. You no longer think of going to the gym as something you *must* do, or your new diet as something you *must* eat. Instead, the new habits become a welcome way of life, an essential part of who you are. This is because you begin to notice small changes, physically and/or psychologically, which are motivating and make you want to continue.

The Primal Body Program is not difficult—you can commit to it for at least six weeks, letting yourself be drawn in to a new way of living life. Anyone can do it and achieve the birthright benefits of *Your Primal Body*.

How about you?

Appendix A: Primal Resources

La Chamba cookware for the ancestral diet
www.mytoque.com

Slimguide Body Fat Caliper
www.fitnesstransform.com/store/

High-Density Foam Roller
www.fitnesstransform.com/store/

The Grid
www.PerformBetter.com

Glycemic index/load
www.mendosa.com/gilists.htm

Kettlebells
www.dragondoor.com

Paleo information
www.paleodiet.com
www.robbwolf.com
www.arthurdevany.com

Nutrition information
www.nutritiondata.self.com/

Appendix B:
Bibliography and Recommended Books

Boyle, Michael. *Functional Training for Sports.* Human Kinetics, 2004.

Cordain, Loren, PhD. *The Paleo Diet: Lose Weight and Get Healthy by Eating the Foods You Were Designed to Eat.* John Wiley & Sons, 2002.

De Vany, Arthur. *The New Evolution Diet: What Our Paleolithic Ancestors Can Teach Us About Weight Loss, Fitness, and Aging.* Rodale, 2010.

Eades, Michael, MD, and Mary Dan Eades, MD. *The Protein Power Lifeplan: A New Comprehensive Blueprint for Optimal Health.* Grand Central Publishing, 2000.

Gedgaudas, Nora T. *Primal Body, Primal Mind: Beyond the Paleo Diet for Total Health and a Longer Life.* Healing Arts Press, 2011.

Keith, Lierre. *The Vegetarian Myth: Food, Justice, and Sustainability.* PM Press, 2009.

Price, Weston A., DDS. *Nutrition and Physical Degeneration.* Price Pottenger Nutrition, 1939; 8th edition, 2008.

Ryan, Christopher, and Cacilda Jetha. *Sex at Dawn: How We Mate, Why We Stray, and What It Means for Modern Relationships.* HarperCollins, 2010.

Taubes, Gary. *Good Calories, Bad Calories: Challenging the Conventional Wisdom on Diet, Weight Control, and Disease.* Alfred A. Knopf, 2007.

——*Why We Get Fat: And What to Do About It.* Alfred A. Knopf, 2011.

Tsatsouline, Pavel. *Enter The Kettlebell! Strength Secret of the Soviet Supermen.* Dragon Door Publications, 2006.

Endnotes

CHAPTER 1

1. "Unearthing Prehistoric Tumors, and Debate," *New York Times,* December 28, 2010.

2. S. B. Eaton and L. Cordain, "Evolutionary Health Promotion: A Consideration of Common Counter-Arguments," *Preventive Medicine* 34 (2002): 119–23; L. Cordain, R. W. Gotshall, and S. B. Eaton, "Physical Activity, Energy Expenditure and Fitness: An Evolutionary Perspective," *International Journal of Sports Medicine* 19, no. 5 (1998): 328–35.

CHAPTER 2

1. Richard D. Feinman et al., "Thermodynamics and Metabolic Advantage of Weight Loss Diets," *Metabolic Syndrome and Related Disorders* 1, no. 3 (2003).

2. Michael R. Eades, MD, www.proteinpower.com/drmike.

3. S. Boyd Eaton, Loren Cordain, and Phillip B. Sparling, "Evolution, Body Composition, Insulin Receptor Competition, and Insulin Resistance," *Preventive Medicine* 49 (2009): 283–85.

4. According to studies on exercise afterburn from a review by Dr. Len Kravitz and Chantal A. Vella, heavy resistance training elicits greater EPOC, when compared to aerobic cycling, lower intensity circuit training, and low-intensity aerobic exercise. Elliot et al. (1988) studied the difference in EPOC between aerobic cycling (40 minutes at 80 percent heart rate max), circuit training (4 sets, 8 exercises, 15 reps at 50 percent 1RM), and heavy resistance training (3 sets, 8 exercises, 3 to 8 reps at 80 to 90 percent 1RM) and found that heavy resistance training produced the greatest EPOC, compared with circuit training and cycling. Gilette et al. (1994) compared resistance training (5 sets, 10 exercises, 8 to 12 reps at 70 percent 1RM) to aerobic exercise (50 percent VO2 max for 60 minutes) and found that the resistance training produced a significantly greater EPOC response. Thornton and Potteiger (2002) compared the effects of a high-intensity (2 sets, 8 reps, 85 percent 8RM) to low-intensity (2 sets, 15 reps, 45 percent 8RM) resistance training and found a significantly greater EPOC with the high-intensity program.

But high-intensity resistance training is not the only way to elicit EPOC. High-intensity interval training produces a significant afterburn, as well. Laforgia et al. (1997) compared the effects of a continuous run (30 minutes at 70 percent VO2 max) to an interval run (20 bouts of 1-minute duration at 105 percent VO2 max) and found significantly greater EPOC following the intermittent bouts of exercise. Kaminski et al. (1990) also found significantly greater EPOC in comparing an intermittent bout of exercise (two 25-minute sessions at 75 percent VO2 max) to a continuous bout of exercise (50-minute continuous run at 75 percent VO2 max).

CHAPTER 3

1. "Glucose Restriction to Enhance Longevity," http://www.sciencedaily.com/releases/2009/12/091217183053.htm.

2. R. Anson et al., "Intermittent Fasting Dissociates Beneficial Effects of Dietary Restriction on Glucose Metabolism and Neuronal Resistance to Injury from Calorie Intake" (2003), http://www.pnas.org/content/100/10/6216.full.

3. F.W. Booth, "Exercise and Gene Expression: Physiological Regulation of the Human Genome Through Physical Activity" (2002), http://jp.physoc.org/content/543/2/399.full.

4. "The Incredible Flying Nonagenarian" http://www.nytimes.com/2010/11/28/magazine/28athletes-t.html?pagewanted=all.

5. Simon Melov et al., "Resistance Exercise Reverses Aging in Human Skeletal Muscle" (2007).

6. See Stevo Ledbetter, http://coachstevo.com/blog/2010/3/16/hard-style-kettlebells-and-benefits-for-female-sexual-respon.html.

CHAPTER 4

1. Greg Wadley and Angus Martin, "The Origins of Agriculture: A Biological Perspective and a New Hypothesis," *Australian Biologist* (June 1993): 96–105, http://ranprieur.com/readings/origins.html.

2. G. D. Brinkworth et al., "Long-Term Effects of a Very-Low-Carbohydrate Weight Loss Diet Compared with an Isocaloric Low-Fat Diet After 12 Months," *American Journal of Clinical Nutrition* (July 2009): 23–32.

3. Michael R. Eades, www.proteinpower.com/drmike.

4. E. L. Knight et al., "The Impact of Protein Intake on Renal Function Decline in Women with Normal Renal Function or Mild Renal Insufficiency," *Annals of Internal Medicine* (March 2003): 460–467; J. R. Poortmans et al., "Do Regular High Protein Diets Have Potential Health Risks on Kidney Function in Athletes?" *International Journal of Sport Nutrition* (March 2000): 28–38.

CHAPTER 5

1. S. B. Eaton, S. B. Eaton III, and M. J. Konner, "Paleolithic Nutrition Revisited: Twelve Year Retrospective on Its Nature and Implications," *European Journal of Clinical Nutrition* 51 (1997): 207–16.

2. Y. Li, C. Wang, K. Zhu, et al., "Effects of Multivitamin and Mineral Supplementation on Adiposity, Energy Expenditure and Lipid Profiles in Obese Chinese Women," *International Journal of Obesity* (London) 34, no. 6 (June 2010): 1070–77; February 9, 2010, http://www.ncbi.nlm.nih.gov/pubmed/20142823.

3. Gedgaudas, *Primal Body, Primal Mind,* 109.

4. Workshop "The Essentiality of and Recommended Dietary Intakes for Omega-6 and Omega-3 Fatty Acids," held in Bethesda, Maryland, and reported in the *Journal of the American College of Nutrition* 18, no. 5, (1999): 487–89, http://www.jacn.org/cgi/content/full/18/5/487.

5. Kelly L. Weaver, Priscilla Ivester, Michael C. Seeds, L. Douglas Case, Jonathan Arm, and Floyd H. Chilton, et al., "Omega Fatty Acid Balance Can Alter Immunity and Gene Expression," *Journal of Biological Chemistry* 284 (June 5, 2009): 15,400–07, http://www.jbc.org/content/284/23/15400.abstract; http://www.eurekalert.org/pub_releases/2009–05/asfb-ofa052909.php.

6. See http://www.westonaprice.org/fat-soluble-activators/miracle-of-vitamin-d.

7. See http://www.vitamindcouncil.org/.

CHAPTER 7

1. Michael Boyle, *Functional Training for Sports* (Place:: Publisher, Year), Page#.

2. Paul Chek, http://www.chekinstitute.com.

CHAPTER 8

1. E. G. Trapp, and S. H. Boutcher, "Fat Loss Following 15 Weeks of High Intensity, Intermittent Cycle Ergometer Training," University of South Wales, Sydney, Australia, 2007.

2. M. D. Schuenke, R. P. Mikat, and J. M. McBride, "Effect of an Acute Period of Resistance Exercise on Excess Post-Exercise Oxygen Consumption: Implications for Body Mass Management," *European Journal of Applied Physiology* 86 (2002): 411–17.

3. I. Tabata, K. Nishimura, M. Kouzaki, et al., "Effects of Moderate-Intensity Endurance and High-Intensity Intermittent Training on Anaerobic Capacity and VO2 Max," *Medicine and Science in Sports and Exercise* 28, no. 10 (1996): 1327–30.

4. Ryan E. Farrar, Jerry L. Mayhew, and Alexander J. Koch, "Oxygen Cost of Kettlebell Swings," *Journal of Strength & Conditioning Research* 24 no. 4 (April 2010): 1034–36.

CHAPTER 11

1. See S. P. Nicolaï et al., "Supervised Exercise Versus Non-Supervised Exercise for Reducing Weight in Obese Adults," *Journal of Sports and Medical Physical Fitness* 49, no. 1 (March 2009): 85–90.

Acknowledgments

I wish to thank my clients, first and foremost, who have shared this fitness journey with me. Thank you for trusting me with your body and your fitness. Working with you has given me the experience that enabled me to write this book. Thanks, too, for those who have let me share their stories in this book.

Thank you to Art De Vany for writing his essay, "Evolutionary Fitness" (1995), which greatly inspired me and completely transformed my thinking on health and fitness.

Thank you to my editor, Nancy Marriott, for showing me how to develop my ideas into a book and for getting it into the hands of my agent. This book would not have happened without your help.

Many thanks to my agent David Nelson at Waterside for finding a great publishing home for my book, Perseus Books.

To my editor at Perseus, Renée Sedliar, and the folks at Da Capo Press, thank you for transforming my manuscript into a book and getting it onto bookshelves everywhere.

Thank you to my model, Tawnnie Pingle, who literally walked into my studio when I was wondering where to find a fitness model for photos.

Thank you to my fellow fitness professionals and associates. I have learned a great deal from all of you along the way. Some of you are mentioned in this book.

And to my mom, Cecelia Reilly, who encouraged me to get an education. Thank you for all your support.

Conversion Chart

General Formula for Metric Conversion

Ounces to grams	Multiply ounces by 28.35
Grams to ounces	Multiply grams by 0.035
Pounds to grams	Multiply pounds by 453.5
Pounds to kilograms	Multiply pounds by 0.45
Cups to liters	Multiply cups by 0.24
Fahrenheit to Celsius	Subtract 32 from Fahrenheit temperature, multiply by 5, divide by 9
Celsius to Fahrenheit	Multiply Celsius temperature by 9, divide by 5, add 32

Volume (Dry) Measurements

¼ teaspoon = 1 milliliter
½ teaspoon = 2 milliliters
¾ teaspoon = 4 milliliters
1 teaspoon = 5 milliliters
1 tablespoon = 15 milliliters
¼ cup = 59 milliliters
⅓ cup = 79 milliliters

½ cup = 118 milliliters
⅔ cup = 158 milliliters
¾ cup = 177 milliliters
1 cup = 225 milliliters
4 cups or 1 quart = 1 liter
½ gallon = 2 liters
1 gallon = 4 liters

Volume (Liquid) Measurements

1 teaspoon = ⅙ fluid ounce = 5 milliliters
1 tablespoon = ½ fluid ounce = 15 milliliters
2 tablespoons = 1 fluid ounce = 30 milliliters
¼ cup = 2 fluid ounces = 60 milliliters
⅓ cup = 2⅔ fluid ounces = 79 milliliters
½ cup = 4 fluid ounces = 118 milliliters
1 cup or ½ pint = 8 fluid ounces = 250 milliliters
2 cups or 1 pint = 16 fluid ounces = 500 milliliters
4 cups or 1 quart = 32 fluid ounces = 1,000 milliliters
1 gallon = 4 liters

Oven Temperature Equivalents
Fahrenheit (F) and Celsius (C)

100°F = 38°C
200°F = 95°C
250°F = 120°C
300°F = 150°C
350°F = 180°C
400°F = 205°C
450°F = 230° C

Linear Measurements

½ inch = 1⅓ cm
1 inch = 2½ cm
6 inches = 15 cm
8 inches = 20 cm
10 inches = 25 cm
12 inches = 30 cm
20 inches = 50 cm

Weight (Mass) Measurements

1 ounce = 30 grams
2 ounces = 55 grams
3 ounces = 85 grams
4 ounces = ¼ pound = 125 grams
8 ounces = ½ pound = 240 grams
12 ounces = ¾ pound = 375 grams
16 ounces = 1 pound = 454 grams

About the Author

Professional certified fitness trainer Mikki Reilly has been teaching people about fitness for twenty years. A one-time competing bodybuilder, she brings her wealth of experience to helping people of all ages lose weight and become fit.

Mikki graduated from the University of California at Santa Barbara with degrees in both exercise and health science, and communication. She earned the highly esteemed certified strength and conditioning specialist (CSCS) credential from the National Strength and Conditioning Association (NSCA) and the master of fitness sciences (MFS) from the International Sports Sciences Association (ISSA).

Mikki was awarded the ISSA Distinguished Achievement Award, which signifies placement in the top 1 percent of certified trainers worldwide. *C Magazine*'s January/February 2007 issue named her as one of the top ten fitness gurus in California. She was featured in *The Complete Guide to Fiscal Fitness: The Business Guide for Personal Trainers* published by the ISSA. In addition, she took the Russian Kettlebell Challenge with Pavel Tsatsouline and became RKC certified. Eighteen months later, she was invited back to assist with instructing trainers and coaches in this elite method.

A proponent and practitioner herself of what evolutionary theorists call the "Paleo" approach, Mikki is a trainer who walks her talk. She adopted the Primal Body lifestyle ten years ago and has never looked back. Today, she's a living example of the benefits available and has inspired and trained a long list of clients who have gotten remarkable results from following her diet and exercise recommendations. As a highly certified trainer, working daily with people to support them accomplishing their fitness goals, she has a unique vantage point to see what works and what doesn't. This perspective allows her to tailor her programs to men and women with a variety of goals and conditions in any age group.

Mikki is also an experienced speaker and writer, presenting recently on health and longevity at the Santa Barbara 2009 Women's Festival. Her articles have been published in *Santa Barbara Fitness Magazine*; *Med Fit*, a personal training trade journal for ISSA; and the *Balance Bar Newsletter*. Additionally, she served on the Balance Health Science Advisory Board and on Metrx's World's Best Personal Trainer Advisory Staff.

Mikki lives in Santa Barbara, California, where she owns and operates her own fitness studio, Fitness Transform. When not training clients, she can be found enjoying the outdoors and staying fit by hiking and skating, among other activities.

For more information, please visit www.yourprimalbody.com.

Index